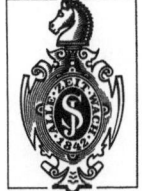

Dierk A. Redel

Color
Blood Flow Imaging
of the Heart

With 214 Figures

Springer-Verlag
Berlin Heidelberg New York
London Paris Tokyo

Prof. Dr. med. DIERK A. REDEL
Universitäts-Kinderklinik
Adenauerallee 119
5300 Bonn

ISBN-13:978-3-642-71174-9   e-ISBN-13:978-3-642-71172-5
DOI: 10.1007/978-3-642-71172-5

Library of Congress Cataloging-in-Publication Data

Redel, Dierk. Color blood flow imaging of the heart / Dierk Redel. p. cm. 1. Doppler echocar-diography. 2. Heart-Imaging. 3. Blood flow-Measurement. 4. Heart-Diseases-Diagnosis. I. Title. [DNLM: 1. Coronary Circulation. 2. Echocardiography-methods. 3. Heart Defects. Congenital-diagnosis.   WG 220 R314c] RC683.5.U5R42 1987 616.07'543-dc 19

© by Springer-Verlag Berlin Heidelberg 1988
Softcover reprint of the hardcover 1st edition 1988

Reproduction of the figures: Gustav Dreher GmbH, Stuttgart
2121/3130-543210

Contents

Preface

Just a very few years after Edler and Hertz had described the clinical use of M-mode echocardiography[1] Satomura reported the application of Doppler ultrasound to the study of cardiac function.[2] Yet Doppler ultrasound has been integrated into diagnostic practice in cardiology much more slowly than conventional (M-mode and two-dimensional) echocardiography. Now, however, tremendous growth in the interest of clinicians in the diagnostic use of Doppler ultrasound can be observed and may in fact be due to the recent advent of color flow imaging. The reason for this growth may be that this method makes it possible to directly visualize the blood flow in the cardiovascular system in cross-sectional views. Moreover, the results are reproducible and much easier to understand than the older mapping techniques using a single-gate Doppler. In its short existence many different names have been used to describe this method, for instance, color Doppler, color flow imaging, real-time two-dimensional Doppler echocardiography, and Doppler flow imaging. This diversity reflects the large interest that many researchers have shown in this method.

The technical development of color blood flow imaging (CBFI) – as this method will be called in this book – has not yet reached a universally accepted standard of performance in cardiology. Despite this state of flux and the uncertainty about future developments, I think it is justified to dedicate an entire book to this fascinating method. Future developments in this field (for instance, digital flow mapping) will not obviate the importance of CBFI.

CBFI is a technique which produces images containing such an unusually high content of densely packed blood flow information that it often cannot be described adequately by words. It has therefore been my aim to present as many different figures as possible for each specific heart disease to enable the reader to view the many different ways in which flow abnormalities can present themselves in one and the same type of cardiovascular abnormality. It is the merit of the staff of Springer-Verlag, especially Mr. B. Lewerich and Dr. U. Heilmann, that they have made my point of view their own and have put much emphasis on a high-quality reproduction of the figures, which had been taken as original photographs from the screen.

The solely technical part of CBFI has intentionally been dealt with very briefly because not much information is available that gives the medically educated and interested reader a comprehensible access to the technological basis of this method. Instead, care has been taken to prepare chapters dealing with the color display of blood flow velocities, with artifacts, and with the display of physiological blood flow patterns in the cardiovascular system.

This book provides optimal profit to the reader who has both experience in the use of two-dimensional echocardiography and some knowledge in the principles of Doppler ultrasound. To facilitate the interpretation of the two-dimensional color flow images the displayed view in each figure has been designated according to the nomenclature of the American Society of Echocardiography Committee. It must, however, be taken into account that in many cases the pathological flow patterns do not obey these standardizing recommendations but have rules of their own. Therefore, it was necessary to modify the orientation of the cross-sectional planes in order to visualize the pathological flow patterns as completely as possible.

I decided not to add schematic drawings to the figures because they have been reproduced in such outstanding quality that this does not seem to be necessary. Instead, the position from which the image has been taken is given in the legend to each figure.

I am indebted to my coworkers and to the technicians of the Department of Pediatric Cardiology at the University of Bonn. These persons include Dr. Wippermann, Dr. Lu and Sonja Seemann. I want also to thank my secretary, Marion Gilessen, for typing most of the manuscript. Last but not least I want to thank everyone who assisted me by word and deed in writing this book.

Bonn, FRG   DIERK A. REDEL
March 3, 1988

[1] Edler I, Hertz CH (1954) Use of ultrasonic reflectoscope with a continuous recording of movements of heart walls. Kung Fysiogr Sallsk Lund Forhand 24: 40–45
[2] Satomura S (1957) Ultrasonic Doppler method for the inspection of cardiac functions. J Acoust Soc Am 29: 1181

1 Introduction

Color blood flow imaging (CBFI) – as this method will be called in the following chapters – is the subject of this book. It is characterized by many fascinating features, which will be shown in a variety of examples and demonstrate that this noninvsive and harmless method can give important diagnostic information. The reliability of its qualitative and semi-quantitative results equals that of the invasive and much more risky method of angiocardiography. Additionally, it offers the option of a comprehensive integration of the various Doppler methods (i.e., single gate pulsed Doppler, continuous wave Doppler) into a very effective diagnostic concept which is easy to understand and quick to learn.

CBFI offers the important advantage that its results are not as limited by subjective interpretations as those of other imaging techniques and are much more elucid than those of conventional Doppler methods. Moreover, CBFI offers quite new insights into the physiology of the cardiovascular system which may, however, lead to interpretational errors as long as we have not had sufficient experience in the use of this method. Therefore, investigations of the normal behavior of blood flow in different age groups and its change under a variety of physiological conditions are one field of research in the next years. In fact, CBFI is ideally suitable for this purpose because investigations can be performed on any human being, including even the fetus, without any known risk. Some results of our studies in this field are presented in Chap. 4.

Concerning the interpretation of CBFI findings in individuals with suspected heart disease, it is important to realize that this method offers information which is quite different from that given by angiocardiography. In the latter the image is based on the opacification by contrast medium; its density is proportional to the magnitude of volume flow. In CBFI the spatial (or temporal) distribution of kinetic energy of blood cells is the relevant parameter. Therefore, these methods may offer divergent findings in extreme situations such as when a small volume of blood is driven by a large pressure gradient causing high flow velocities or when a large blood volume is driven by a relatively small pressure difference. The former situation can be found in critical valvular stenoses or in small regurgitations of the left-sided valves while the latter may be encountered in severe valvular regurgitations or in large ventricular septal defects with pulmonary hypertension.

Artifacts may be a severe drawback in any diagnostic method and may induce diagnostic errors if they are not given adequate consideration. A whole chapter (Chap. 3) has been dedicated to this phenomenon in CBFI.

The technology of CBFI is still in its beginnings, which means that there are several limitations with respect to the display of special flow conditions. These include the detection of low velocities as they are normally found in the venous system or as they exist under pathological conditions in low-output states. Some technical solutions of this problem have been proposed and will be referred to later.

The physical phenomenon of aliasing, which is common to all pulsed Doppler systems, may cause confusion in some situations even for the experienced investigator. In other settings, in contrast, it may be helpful for special purposes, such as depicting the spatial (and temporal) distribution fo flow velocities, as will be shown later.

A very important feature of CBFI systems is the display of the variance of frequency shift, which indicates disturbed blood flow. There are several approaches to this point including, unfortunately, differences in color display and the use of different algorithms to define the disturbance itself. This means that the display of blood flow patterns for similar flow situations may be quite different with different CBFI systems and therefore misleading for the investigator. This point will not be settled until the optimal way to detect and display turbulence have been defined.

2 Principles of Color Blood Flow Imaging

The basic principle of color blood flow imaging (CBFI) is based on the Doppler effect, which is valid for the emission as well as for the reflection of energetic waves. The Doppler shift caused by the ultrasound reflection from the corpuscles of the flowing blood is used as a means to investigate blood flow. CBFI utilizes the range-gating properties, i.e., pulsed emission and reception, of ultrasound waves. The pulsed mode leads to the fact that there is a maximal measurable flow velocity for a given transducer frequency under a constant angle; this maximum is caused by the strictly limited maximal pulse repetition frequency (PRF) for a given depth. If blood velocities exceed the maximal measurable value, aliasing occurs (see p. 8).

2.1 Acquisition of Blood Flow Data

Data are collected by processing the irregular Doppler shift signals using the autocorrelation technique [5, 39]. This technique allows very fast determination of the Doppler frequency shift for each sampling point, which takes less time than the propagation of ultrasound from the transducer into the heart and back again. After passing through a quadrature phase detector to determine the direction of phase shift, the echo signal is filtered and fed into the autocorrelator where the determination of the instantaneous phase shift between subsequent pulse trains is performed over all the depths under investigation. In color B-mode this is performed typically for a total number of eight pulses along one sector line. This is the smallest number possible to give sufficient data to achieve an acceptable signal-to-noise ratio and a good differentiation between flow velocities with higher and lower dispersion.

Along each line there are up to 512 points of interest defined over a depth of 18 cm, and for each the detection of the Doppler frequency shift is performed using the fast autocorrelation technique.

Statistical calculations of the flow velocity data are immediately performed in the correlator and yield the mean value and the variance of Doppler-shifted frequencies for each specific sampling point [38].

Table 2.1 Range of frame rates dependent on the color imaging sector angle (Aloka SSD 880)

Frame rate: Maximum: 30 frames per second
30 frames per second at color image angle of 28°
10–30 frames per second at color image angles of 46° and 53°
7.5–15 frames per second at color image angle of 90°
Specific frame rate depends upon pulse repitition frequency

The sector plane is formed by the radial arrangement of 16–64 lines, the number being dependent on the width of the sector angle, and stored in the digital scan converter. The largest angle is 90° and is made up of 64 lines, the smallest is 30° and is made up of 16 lines.

The instantaneous velocity information for each specific sampling point is passed through the color processor and becomes color encoded with respect to flow direction, mean velocity, and variance. This information is displayed on the video screen with a frame rate of between 7.5 frames (90° sector) and 30 frames (30° angle) per second and superimposed on the conventional two-dimensional (2D) image which is presented in white on black.

The time necessary to build up the sector plane varies between 30 ms for the 30° angle sector and 170 ms for the 90° angle sector. Table 2.1 lists the interrelationship between sector angle and frame rate for one of the commercially available systems (Aloka SSD 880).

In the colored M-mode (M/Q-mode) sampling and calculation of velocity data are performed on 64 consecutive echo pulse trains thereby yieding a high spatial density of data over the whole depth under investigation and a good signal-to-noise ratio with a time resolution which is much better than that of the 2D flow image.

2.2 Color Encoding

Blood flow velocity data are color encoded in the digital format by the color processor. At the moment this seems to be the only way to make the large amount of blood flow information immediately available to the investigator. Moreover, color-encoded display of flow velocities offers the unique opportunity of displaying blood flow patterns within the heart and the great vessels [7] exactly where they occur. The structures are displayed in black and white with 64 shades of a gray scale. The information inherent in the Doppler signal is representative of special characteristics of blood flow: an increase in Doppler shift or in phase shift indicates flow towards the transducer and is encoded in red, a decrease indicates flow direction away from the transducer and is imaged in blue (see Fig. 5.12 p. 35,

Fig. 2.1 Normal left ventricular outflow in systole (T1) and inflow in early diastole (T2) imaged in the parasternal long axis view RBG2.
Flow velocities are in the physiological range and do not show any disturbances as can be judged from the lack of green, yellow or aliasing

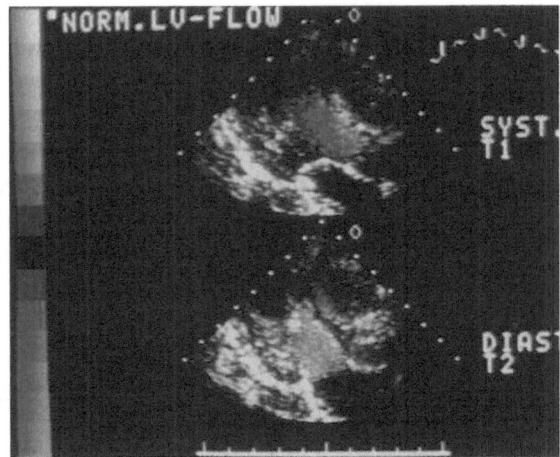

Fig. 3.4a, p. 16). This display mode will be called RB1 on the following pages. The amount of frequency shift is proportional to the velocities of blood flow, their mean values over time are displayed as changes in brightness of red or blue for every specific sampling point (see Fig. 5.3, p. 28, Fig. 5.5a, p. 30, Fig. 5.10, p. 34), it will be called RB2. The variance of flow velocities is a statistical value of their dispersion and an indicator of flow turbulence. It is encoded by adding green to red or blue over a range of 16 steps. Approaching turbulent flow tends towards yellow while receding turbulent flow tends towards turquoise (Fig. 2.2) and will be called RBG2. Low velocities cannot have as high values of variance as high velocities, this fact is displayed in the color bar in Fig. 2.1 where low intensity colors attain less yellow or turquoise than the higher intensities. The dispersion of lower velocities can be demonstrated more clearly if velocity grading is

Fig. 2.2 Severe mitral regurgitation as an example of spatial transition of laminar into turbulent blood flow (RBG2). The M/Q-line is positioned in the central part of the regurgitant jet *(2D insert)* which fills the left atrium almost completely. The M/Q-mode displays the normal left ventricular systolic flow *(blue)* which gradually changes into *turquoise* proximal to the mitral leaflet and splashes through the incompetent valve in a turbulent manner into the left atrium where alias and eddies *(yellow)* appear. Note the much higher density of flow information in the M/Q-mode than in the 2D color image

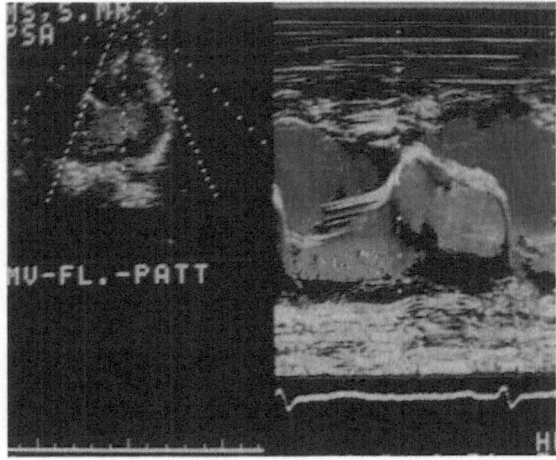

taken off the display (see Fig.6.7, p.48). This, however, results in an un-qualifiable display of relative dispersion with equal brightness over the whole velocity range. On the following pages this mode will be called RBG1.

Figure 2.2 shows the transition of physiological blood flow in the left ventricle (blue) into turbulent blood flow through an incompetent mitral valve (turquoise) with aliasing and the formation of vortices (yellow).

2.3 Color Aliasing

Being necessarily a pulsed Doppler technique, CBFI is liable to aliasing if the frequency shift exceeds the Nyquist limit. This is expressed in a sudden color change in the opposite direction, starting there at the maximal

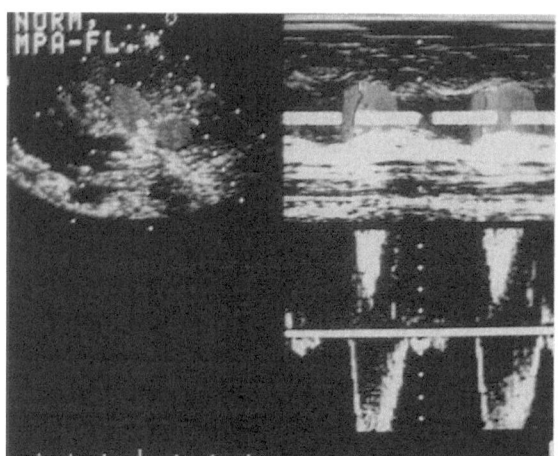

Fig.2.3a, b Examples of color aliasing in the normal main pulmonary artery (RBG2).
a Simultaneous registration of M/Q-mode and single gate Doppler FFT. The sample volume is positioned in the central part of the main pulmonary artery. The actual velocity exceeds the maximal measurable value of 46 cm/s. Aliasing appears at the same time in both modes. Maximal velocity can be measured more accurately in the FFT trace

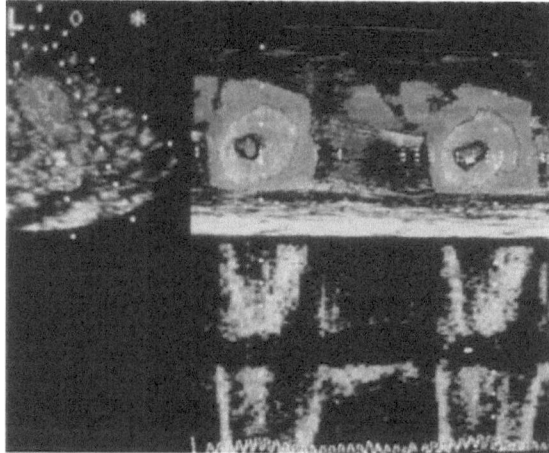

b Simultaneous measurement of M/Q-mode and single gate Doppler, the sample volume is positioned in the central part of the main pulmonary artery *(2-D insert)*. Two fold aliasing is displayed occurring at exactly the same time in the M/Q-mode as well as in the FFT trace velocity display of the opposite color. This is exactly the same as in the single gate Doppler technique with fast Fourier transformed (FFT) spectral analysis (Fig. 2.3 a).

With increasing velocity the opposite color bar is transversed from the top to the bottom, the intensity becoming darker as the velocity increases. If it approaches the two-fold value of the Nyquist limit, the color display arrives at zero. With still further increase, the dark area of zero – which is now double the maximal velocity – is crossed and display starts again at the bottom of the original color bar (Fig. 2.3 b). But this value now has to be added to twice the maximal velocity.

Color aliasing allows the imaging of the spatial distribution of flow velocities over the section of a vessel or a valve. It gives a reproducible definition of flow velocities at the alias points, as can be seen from Fig. 2.3. It may therefore be very useful in determining the spatial distribution of

Fig. 2.4 a, b Normal left ventricular outflow velocities in early systole RBG2. Aliasing occurs in the distal outflow tract near the interventricular septum because flow velocities exceed the Nyquist limit of 92 cm/s, assuming an angle Θ of 0° (a).
Using color baseline shift (b) aliasing is eliminated (see colour bars on the left). *LV*, left ventricle; *LA*, left atrium; *AO*, aorta

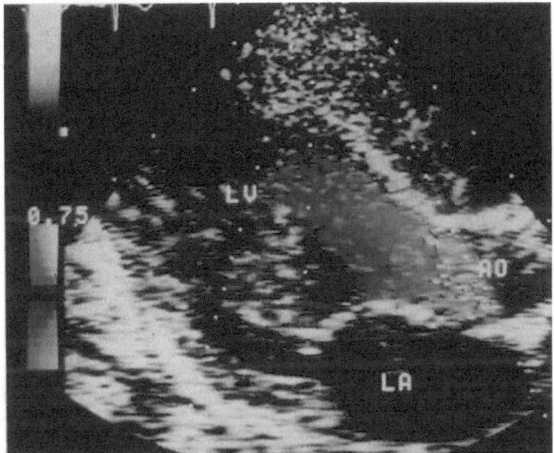

a

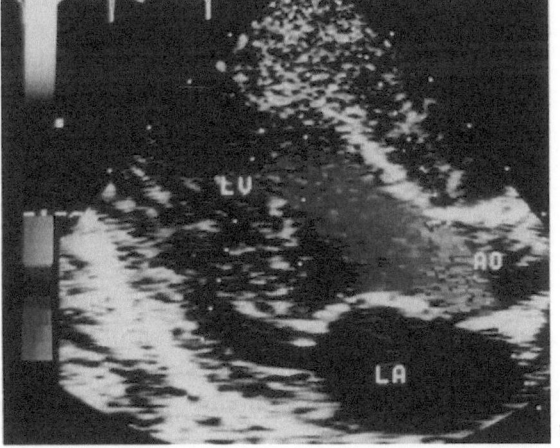

b

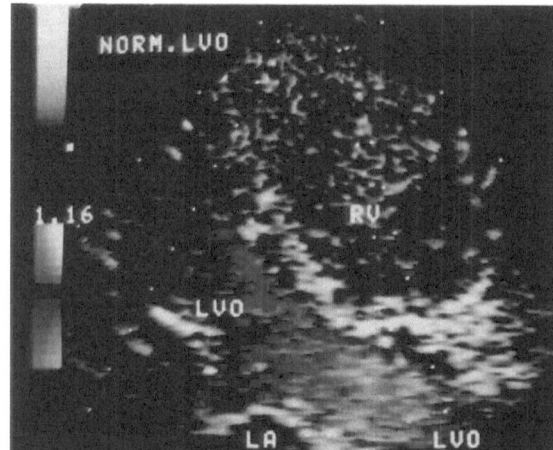

Fig. 2.5 a, b Normal outflow velocities of the left ventricle are below the Nyquist limit of 1.43 m/s, therefore the ventricular outflow *(LVO)* is colored entirely in *blue RBG2.* (a).
However, aliasing can be introduced by moving the color baseline in the away *(blue)* direction (b) and thereby lowering the Nyquist limit. *RV,* right ventricle (see colour bar on the left)

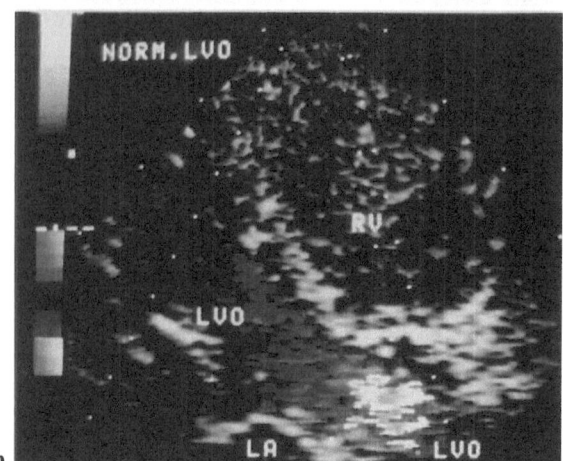

physiological flow profiles over the section of a vessel or a heart chamber at a particular time (isovelocity flow mapping technique). The time component of the flow profile can be displayed in the M/Q-mode, as shown in Fig. 2.3. Moreover, color aliasing may sometimes be very helpful in imaging pathological flow states, i. e., jet-like streaming in valvular or subvalvular stenoses, regurgitations, or in high-pressure shunts, as will be shown later. Imaging of flow velocities is, however, considerably influenced by the choice of PRF. The half value of the PRF determines the frequency level at which aliasing takes place. CBFI is also influenced by the carrier frequency of the transducer according to the Doppler equation, which states that for a given PRF the Nyquist limit decreases in proportion to an increase in carrier frequency. This has to be considered in the pediatric age group when a high-frequency transducer is used in small children or infants.

The alias point can be changed by shifting the baseline up or down as is well known from FFT spectral analysis. Second generation color systems have incorporated this opportunity as a pre- or postprocessing device, thereby enabling the investigator to avoid or to induce aliasing at any desirable point of the velocity scale (Fig. 2.4a + b, 2.5a + b).

2.4 Sensitivity of CBFI

The sensitivity of CBFI is dependent upon the mode of color display (see p. 6). The basic RB1-mode has the highest sensitivity of all modes available, but may be, however, still below that of a single gate Doppler system with FFT spectral analysis (Fig. 2.6a). In this mode blood flow direction is

Fig. 2.6a, b Sensitivity of CBFI demonstrated by left ventricular *(LV)* inflow and outflow in the second fetus of a twin pregnancy in week 25 of pregnancy. Simultaneous recording of color M/Q-mode and single gate Doppler measurement to show the sensitivity of autocorrelation and color encoding as compared the FFT spectral analysis. The *line* within the M/Q-mode indicates the position of the sample volume.
a In the RB1 color display CBFI is nearly as sensitive as FFT spectral analysis

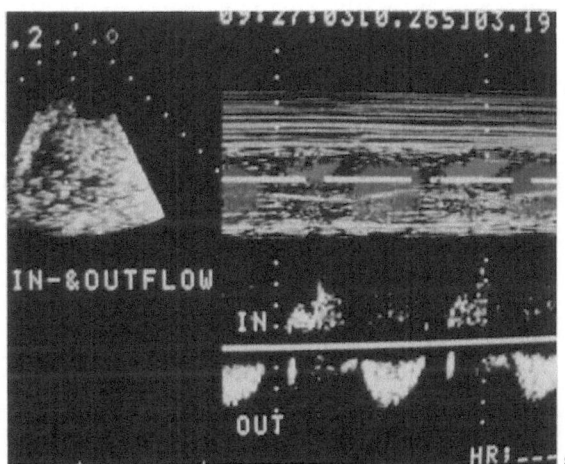

b The RBG2 color display causes decrease in sensitivity by introducing the display of variance. The first diastolic inflow has nearly disappeared from the M/Q-mode whereas the second is imaged as a biphasic pattern

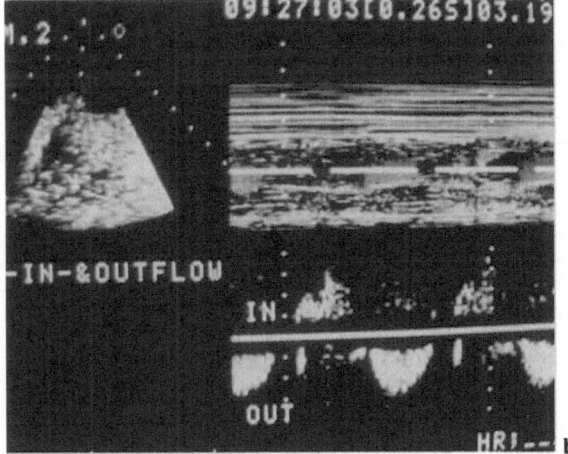

the only information displayed. Various blood flow velocities as well as wall motions are imaged with the same degree of brightness. A similar mode of blood flow display in which the amplitude of the back-scattered echo signal is displayed by different intensities has been implemented into a recently developed color Doppler system and is called "power mode display" [35].

Sensitivity of CBFI decreases slightly if velocity grading is added to the display of flow direction (RB2-mode). The decrease in sensitivity is more pronounced if the display of variance is added by green modulation of blue or red (RBG2-mode), as shown in Fig. 2.6b. There is no difference in sensitivity between the RBG1- and RBG2-modes.

CBFI can be useful for several purposes. Depending on the purpose, certain color display modes may offer specific advantages. For example, if we want to investigate the flow profile across the diameter of the left ventricular inflow tract the RB2-display has proved to be the most useful (see Fig. 5.5 a + b, p. 30). This is because in the RBG2-display there is some visual interference between the velocity encoding brightness and the variance encoding hue which may lead to erroneous impressions, i. e. that velocities are higher at the margin than in the center of the flow area, because in the latter location flow variance is higher than in the center but flow velocities are lower (see Figs. 4.4, p. 24 and 5.16a, p. 38).

3 Artefacts in Color Blood Flow Imaging

Colour blood flow imaging (CBFI) is liable to artefacts in the same way as any ultrasound method. Morever, since CBFI carries the new message of blood flow velocities (and motion of cardiac structures) in a color-encoding display, artefacts are found in a different visual presentation and at unexpected locations.

3.1 Reverberations

Reverberations are caused by reflections of structural echoes at the surface of the transducer [14, p.27]. They are well known from M-mode and 2D echocardiography and they also occur in CBFI. They may affect wall motions [41, p.51] as well as flow velocity areas. In Fig.3.1 the diastolic flow area of the mitral valve and the posterior wall motion appear twice: the anterior area is the real one, the posterior is an artefact caused by reverberation. It shows all the criteria of reverberation: its distance is twice that of the real area and it has a larger and coarser structure. This can be easily avoided if the appropriate depth of penetration is chosen.

Fig.3.1 Reverberation of diastolic mitral valve inflow in the parasternal short axis view (RBG2). Reverberation of the mitral orifice and the wall motion ghost signals behind the heart are shown. It is interesting that the velocity information in the reverberation artefact is lower than that in the real display

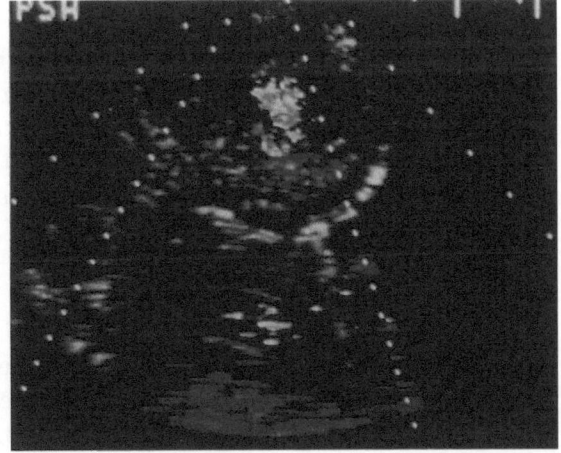

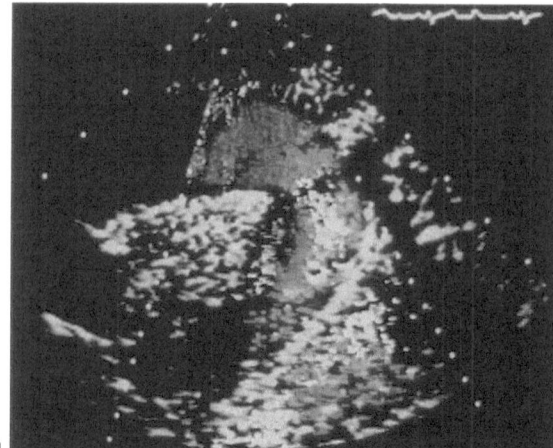

Fig. 3.2 a, b Mirroring displayed behind the descending aorta in the suprasternal long axis view.
a CBFI (RBG2) shows mirroring of the flow display in the distal part of the arch occurring behind the posterior wall of the aorta

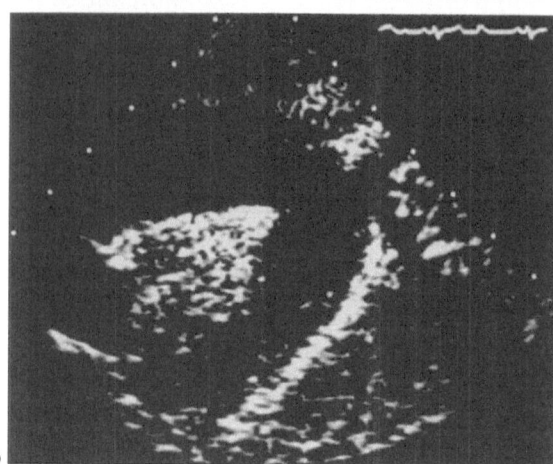

b The 2D image displays only a few structural echoes behind the posterior aortic wall

3.2 Mirroring

Mirroring of flow areas may occur at the walls of the central great vessels. Frequently it is found posterior to the descending aorta in the suprasternal long axis view (Fig. 3.2), here the posterior wall acts as a mirror for ultrasound waves. It is important to know about these artefacts so as not to misdiagnose, for example, an aortic aneurysm.

3.3 Wall Motion Artefacts

The origin of wall motion artefacts is at the moving walls of the heart. They may present themselves as intensively colored echo-reflecting structures because of cardiac contraction. Figure 3.3 a shows the right atrium in

Fig.3.3a, b Wall motion arte-facts.

a Left-to-right shunt *(yellow)* across an atrial septal defect of the secundum type *(ASD II)* in the subcostal four-chamber view (RBG2). The shunt area is encir-cled by wall motion artefacts. See text for more details

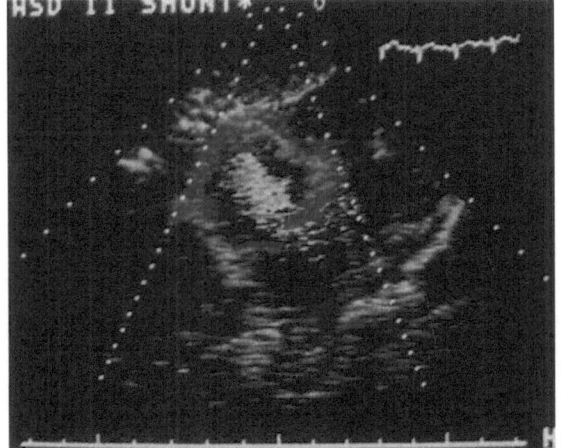

b Early diastolic frame in severe mitral regurgitation in the apical long axis view (RBG2). The rapid expansion of the left ventricle causes intense wall motion arte-facts surrounding early diastolic inflow. Wall motion artefacts can be differentiated from blood flow by their lack of dispersion indicat-ed in this case by a *clear blue col-oration*

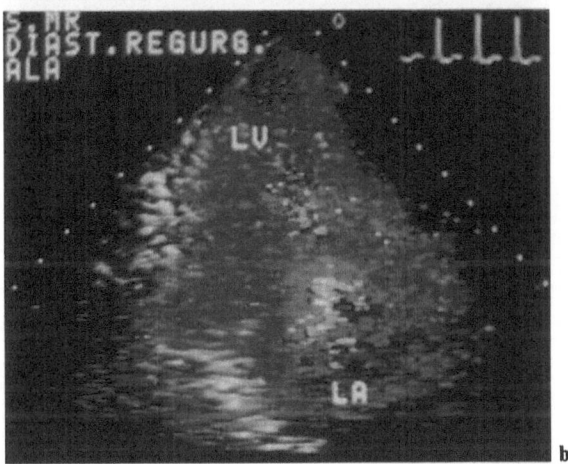

late diastole in a case of atrial septal defect in the subcostal four-chamber view. The yellow area in the right atrium represents the left-to-right shunt. The blue coloration of the walls of the right atrium is caused by the dia-stolic expansion of the right atrium in which the diaphragm is used as a hypomochlion. Much stronger wall motion artefacts with multiple rever-berations, called "wall motion ghost signals", are caused by the walls of the left ventricle in hyperkinetic states [71]. Figure 3.3b shows such strong wall motion ghost signals in early diastole in a case of severe mitral regur-gitation of rheumatic origin. The strong wall artefacts almost completely overshadow the blood flow signals at this moment of rapid ventricular ex-pansion.

In the M/Q-mode wall motion artefacts can be very disturbing (Fig.3.4a). As can be seen in Fig.3.4b they are less pronounced in the RBG2-mode.

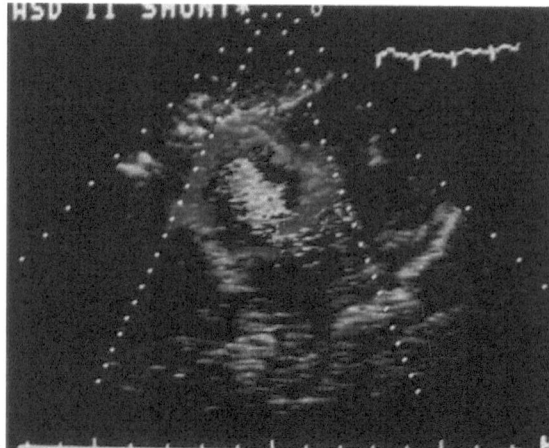

Fig. 3.4a, b M/Q-mode of aortic root blood flow. Abrupt color change is caused by an inappropriate high parasternal transducer position.

a In the RB1 color display *red* immediately changes to *blue* as flow direction changes with the motion of the aortic root. Wall motions cannot be differentiated from flow

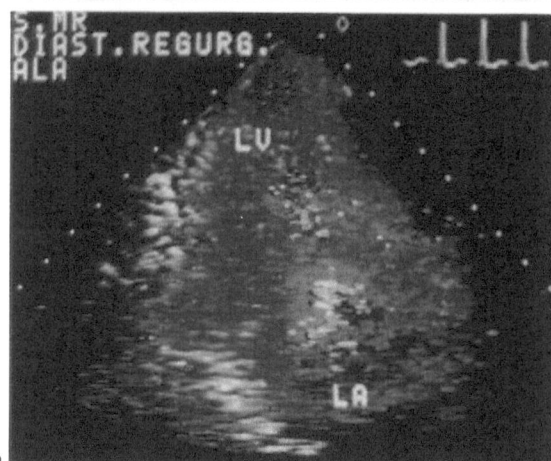

b The RBG2 color display represents a much higher level of signal processing by displaying each Doppler signal according to its frequency, height, and dispersion. Forward and reverse flow in the aortic root are divided by a small region of zero flow. Wall motions are practically eliminated because of their low Doppler shift and narrow spectral bandwidth

These artefacts can be minimized by setting the Doppler pulse repetition frequency as high as possible and by looking at the heart at different time periods when the walls move less rapidly. Additionally, a certain amount of suppression can be obtained by chosing the RBG2-mode.

In second generation CBFI systems a digital "wipe"-function is used eliminating the color from all structures displayed in black and white by introducing tissue priority. In Figure 3.5 there is an example of this function. It shows the right atrium in diastole; in Figure 3.5a blood is flowing, towards the transducer (yellow-orange). Wall motion causes the myocardial structures and the surrouding tissue to become colored. In Figure 3.5b tissue priority is activated. Color is wiped out wherever a structure is displayed in black and white.

In flow conditions where small jets are surrounded by tissue structures, as in small ventricular septal defects, high degree stenoses or in mild val-

Fig. 3.5 a, b Right atrium viewed in the subcostal long axis view. Two-dimensional image of the cavity of the right atrium with the superposition of CBFI (RBG2) (**a**) visualizes the blood flow in the right atrium coming mainly from the superior vena cava *(yellow)* in this section. However, superposition of CBFI also introduces wall motion artefacts which cause coloration of the surrounding tissue. By activating tissue priority function (**b**), color is "wiped out" in all locations which show tissue structures *(black and white)*

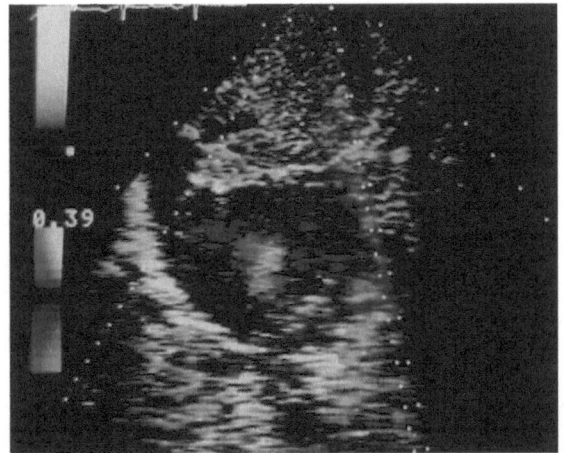

a

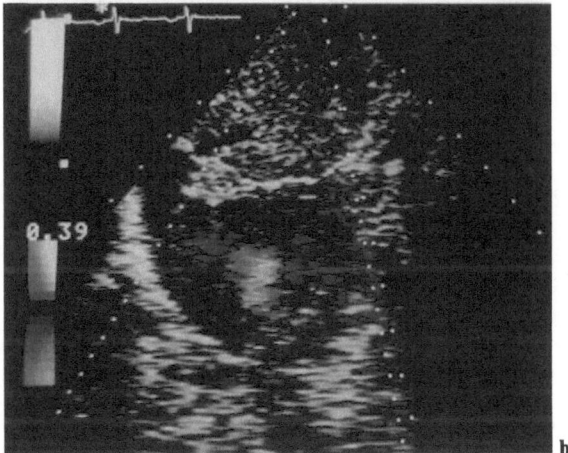

b

vular regurgitations, tissue priority may, however, eliminate the passage of flow through the structures (Fig. 3.6).

3.4 Inappropriate Transducer Position

An inappropriate transducer position for investigation may lead to an abrupt change of flow direction due to the motion of the cardiovascular structures. This may happen if the transducer is positioned nearly perpendicular to the structure under investigation. Figure 3.4 shows such an artefact in the aortic root caused by a parasternal position which is too high, so that the angle between transducer beam and blood flow direction is nearly 90° and causes a change in flow direction in midsystole.

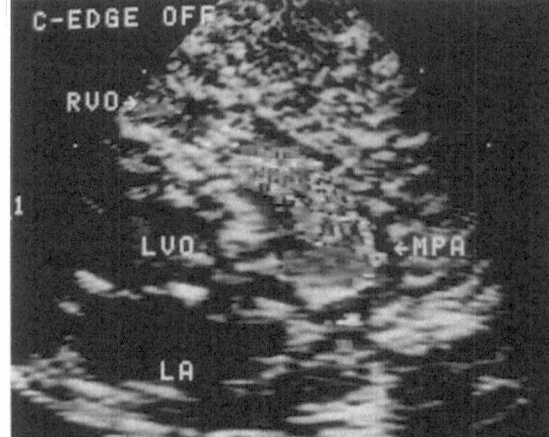

Fig. 3.6a, b Systolic jet in moderately severe pulmonic stenosis.
a The jet can be clearly seen to pass through the thickened pulmonic valves from the right ventricular outflow tract *(RVO)* into the main pulmonary artery *(MPA)*

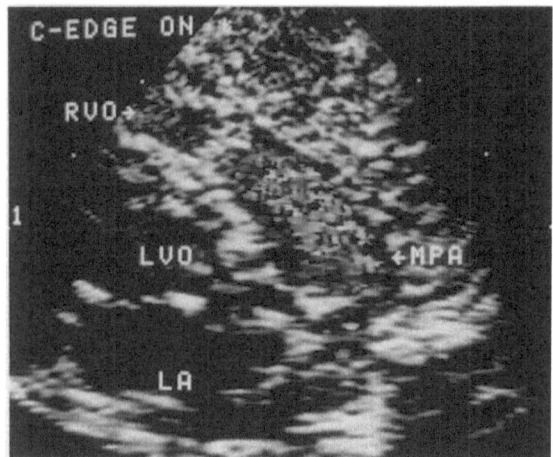

b Activation of tissue priority causes the jet through the stenotic pulmonic orifice to be "wiped out." Without knowing **a**, this could be misdiagnosed as pulmonary valve atresia with perfusion of MPA through a persistent ductus arteriosus

3.5 Distortion of Flow Velocity Display

A distortion of flow phenomena in the 2D image may be caused by the build-up time of the sector (time distortion). Figure 3.7 shows the jet of an incompetent mitral valve splashing into the left atrium. A considerable twisting of the jet is recognizable at its distal part. This bending of the jet can be explained by the time period needed to build up the sector image. During this time the jet has changed its direction owing to the motion of the atrioventricular valve level caused by ventricular contraction. In this special case it takes about 66 ms to build up the sector so that there is a time lag of about 30 ms between the build-up of the head and the tail of the jet. During this time period a change in jet direction has occurred and has caused the jet to bend.

Fig. 3.7 Time distortion in mitral regurgitation, modified parasternal short axis view (RBG2). The twisting of the regurgitant jet is caused by the build-up time of the image. See text for more details

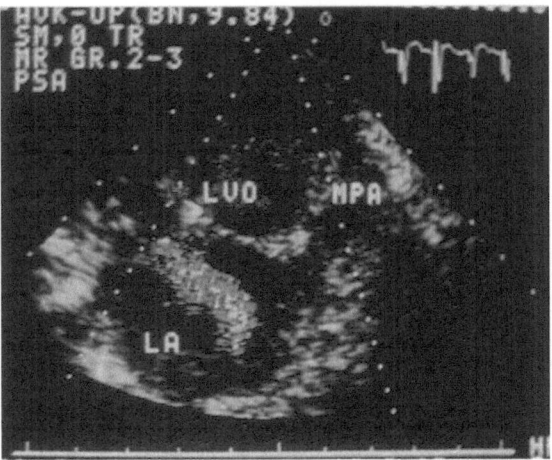

Second generation CBFI systems usually have high frame rates combined with high Doppler PRFs for low penetration depths so that the rapidly beating hearts of infants and children can be imaged more appropriately without the disturbing artefacts caused by time distortion.

3.6 Azimuth Artefacts

The scan plane thickness (azimuth) is different in a 2D image and CBFI. This is, however, not surprising since the two imaging processes are completely different in respect to their physical origin and to the gain level used for echo amplification. CBFI takes place on a much higher level of echo amplification than conventional 2D imaging (about 40 dB). This

Fig. 3.8 Superposition of left ventricular outflow upon the 2D image of a ventricular septal defect *(VSD)* of a fetus in week 27 of pregnancy (RB1). Misinterpretation of left ventricular-right atrial shunt may be caused by the different sector plane thickness (azimuth) of the 2 echocardiographic and the CBFI image. See text for more details. *RA,* right atrium

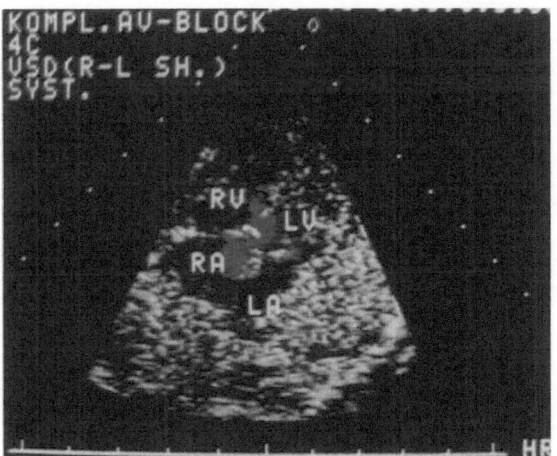

leads of necessity to a greater dimension of the flow imaging plane than of the 2D plane in the x-axis. Figure 3.8 shows an example of the divergence of the two imaging planes in respect to the azimuth: in addition to the right-to-left shunt through the perimembranous ventricular septal defect there seems to be a shunt from the left ventricle into the right atrium. After birth, however, the latter finding could not be confirmed. Therefore it seems reasonable to assume that the left-ventricular right-atrial shunt was simulated by the normal systolic outflow into the aorta, which was displayed by the greater azimuth of the CBFI sector and then superimposed on the 2D image.

4 Color Display of Blood Flow Velocities

This chapter will describe typical color images of various kinds of flow characteristics. This forms the basis for recognizing and understanding the pathological flow conditions in different forms of heart disease. As will be seen, there are only a few archetypical flow patterns and the knowledge of these will make the recognition of pathological states much easier.

4.1 Physiological Flow with Flat Profile

Physiological flow with a flat profile is found in only a few areas of the heart and the central great arteries. These are mainly the atrioventricular valves during diastolic filling in normal or low-flow states (see Fig. 5.5 a, p. 30). In high-flow states, for example, during physical activity, anemia, or left-to-right shunt, a parabolic flow profile across the diameter is observed even in the orifices of the atrioventricular valves or the outflow tracts of the cardiac chambers (see Fig. 5.17, p. 39).

4.2 Physiological Flow with Non-Flat Profile

Physiological flow with a non-flat profile is found in most areas of the heart and the central great arteries. It consists of a nonhomogeneous distribution of flow vectors across the radial and along the longitudinal axis of inflow and outflow tracts. Figure 2.3 (p. 8) shows the spatial distribution and time course of flow vectors within the pulmonary artery of healthy subjects. Our group published a paper in which the flow profile in the main pulmonary artery (MPA) was studied in 50 children [53]. A reasonably flat profile was found in only two of them, 48 individuals exhibited an nonhomogeneous distribution of flow velocity vectors across and along the MPA. It consisted of higher velocities in blood flow in the center than near the walls or in the proximal or distal parts of MPA. In 22 children the central velocities were more than two-fold higher during more than one-quarter of systole (see Fig. 2.3). For more details concerning the distribution of velocities see Table 4.1 and Fig. 4.1.

Table 4.1.

50 pat	Group A	Group B	Group C
A A (cm/s)	< 46	< 46	< 46
R B1 (cm/s)	< 46	46 < V > 69	69 < V > 92
E B2 (cm/s)	46 < V > 69	69 < V > 92	> 92
A B3 (cm/s)	< 46	< 46	69 < V > 92
S C (cm/s)	< 46	46 < V > 69	46 < V > 69
n	3	24	23
L-R shunt	0	9	10

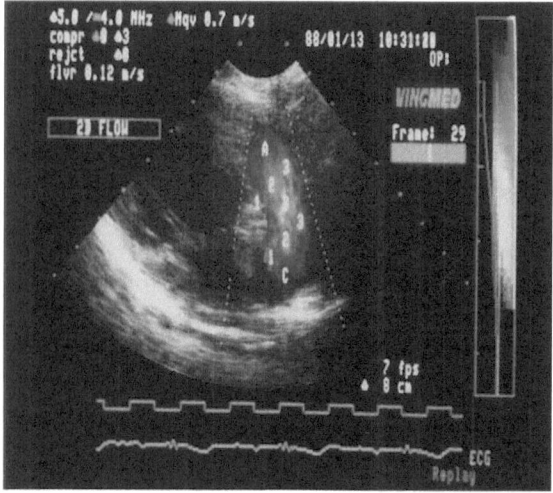

Fig. 4.1 In our study (53) the pulmonary artery has been divided into three longitudinal (A to C) and into three transversal (1 to 3) areas. The range of blood flow velocities in the MPA has been determined by judging the phenomenon of aliasing at three different pulse repetition frequencies in each one of the above mentioned areas. Colour reversal indicated that a certain velocity was exceeded which equaled 92 cm/s in the PRF-range of 8 KHz, 69 cm/s in the 6 KHz mode and 46 cm/s using a PRF of 4 KHz with a 3.5 MHz transducer the angle of investigation being about 0 degrees. The determined velocities were written down for each of the abovementioned areas in 50 children, the numerical results of which are shown in table 4.1. They indicate that in only three of the 50 individuals the flow profile could not be observed to be assymmetric because blood flow did not exceed the level of twofold aliasing

4.3 Convective Acceleration

Convective acceleration is found under *physiological* conditions in the inflow and outflow tracts of the ventricles. It is caused by the diminishing cross section of the cardiac chambers towards the valves and is especially pronounced below the arterial valves. It is easy to be imaged below the

Fig. 4.2 Systolic convective acceleration in the left ventricle towards the incompetent mitral valve in severe mitral regurgitation. Left ventricular *(LV)* blood is flowing away from the transducer towards the base of the heart and velocity is increasing towards the incompetent mitral valve. Turbulence *(turquoise)* and alias *(yellow)* are visible in front of the mitral valve and indicate pathological convective acceleration

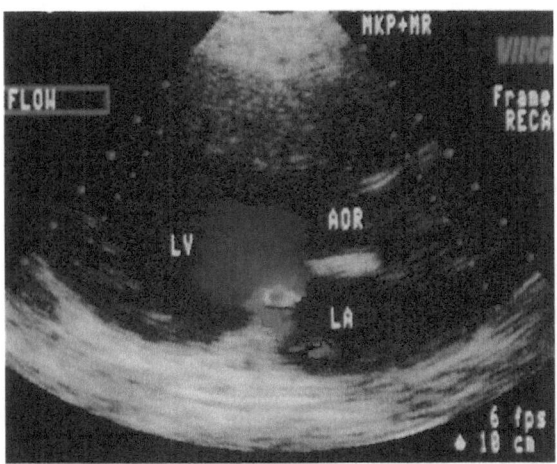

aortic valve in the long axis view because of the straight course of the left ventricular outflow tract where it is recognizable by an increase in color brightness (see Fig. 2.1, p. 7, Fig. 2.5a, p. 10) or by aliasing (Fig. 2.4a, p. 9, 2.5b, p. 10). Convective acceleration towards the pulmonic valve is much more difficult to visualize because the inflow and outflow of the right ventricle are separated and the latter takes a curved course. In *pathological* conditions convective acceleration (venae contractae) is seen proximal to stenoses (Fig. 4.2) regurgitations (see Fig. 2.2, p. 7), or shunting defects (see Fig. 6.14b, p. 55), when considerable pressure differences are found between the proximal and distal sites of the narrowing. In addition to increasing brightness or aliasing as hallmarks of rising flow velocities, there is often a more or less green modulation as an indicator of the appearance of flow disturbance proximal to the regurgitant site (Fig. 4.2).

4.4 Streamline Separation

Streamline separation is the appearance of flow velocities having orthograde and retrograde directions in one vessel at the same time. We have observed this phenomenon in the great arteries in a variety of conditions and studied it in the pulmonary artery in pulmonary hypertension [49, 54], in idiopathic ectasia of the pulmonary artery (Fig. 4.3), and after surgical correction of heart diseases as for instance defects with left-to-right shunt or pulmonary valve stenosis [83]. The denominator common to all of these conditions is a considerable dilatation of the MPA which causes a separation of streams of the outflowing blood at the inferior wall of the pulmonary artery, which in return produces backflow from the bifurcation towards the right ventricular outflow tract [82]. If this backflow is

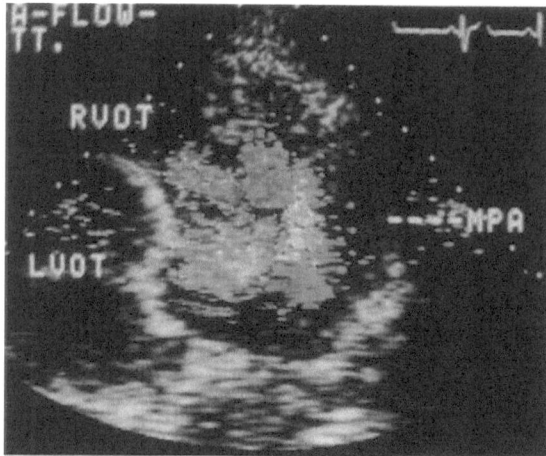

Fig. 4.3 Systolic streamline separation in the main pulmonary artery *(MPA)*, parasternal long axis view of MPA (RBG2). Blood is flowing back *(orange-yellow)* from the bifurcation towards the right ventricular outflow tract *(RVOT)* at the inferior wall above the left ventricular outflow tract *(LVOT)*

pronounced, it may reach the posterior pulmonary valve leaflet and may lead to a systolic closing movement, called "systolic notching" of the pulmonic valve [80]. The same phenomenon is responsible for mesosystolic notching of the aortic valve in discrete subaortic stenosis (see p. 92).

4.5 Angle Dependency of CBFI

The cosine function of the angle Θ is one of the proportionality factors in the Doppler equation for calculating the flow velocities from the Doppler-shifted frequencies. Therefore, CBFI as a Doppler technique is angle dependent. Arterial flow velocities are nevertheless imaged up to an angle of nearly 90°, as can be seen in Fig. 4.4. This figure shows systolic flow veloc-

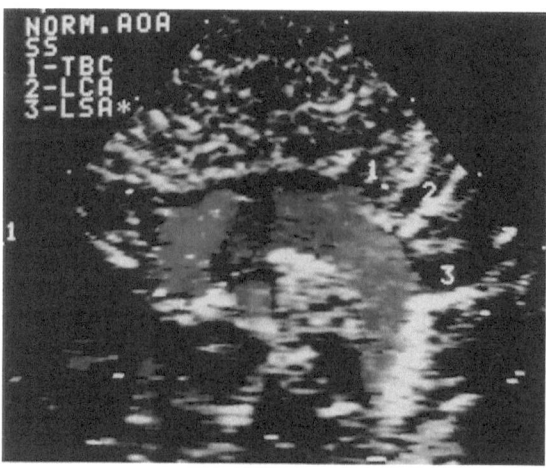

Fig. 4.4 Normal systolic flow velocities in the aorta, viewed from the suprasternal position (RBG2). The influence of direction and of the ange Θ on the velocity display is shown. In the ascending aorta *(AOA, red-orange)*, the aortic arch *(dark blue)* and the descending aorta *(light blue)*, blood flow velocities are in the same range. However, the difference in direction and angle 0 caused by the bending of the aortic arch leads to a continuous difference of the frequency shifts in the different parts of the aorta. See text for more details. *1,* brachiocephalic trunc; *2,* left common carotid artery; *3,* left subclavian artery

ities in the aortic arch from the suprasternal position. In the proximal part, flow is directed towards the transducer and displayed in red-yellow, in the distal parts and at the beginning of the descending aorta, blood is flowing away from the transducer and is imaged in blue. The continuous change of the angle Θ produced by the curvature of the aortic arch leads to a representation of equal velocities along the aorta by continuously changing Doppler frequencies, as can be seen from the continuous increase in color brightness in the descending aorta caused by a decrease in angle Θ.

4.6 Disturbed Flow

Turbulence occurs in high velocities if the Reynold's number is exceeded. As a rule, this happens in pathological flow conditions. It is characterized by a broadened spectrum of velocities being found in one area and is displayed by a dispersion of Doppler frequencies. Dispersion is dealt with statistically by an increase in variance. In CBFI variance is expressed by adding green to the primary two colors red and blue in several steps according to the degree of dispersion (p. 7). If flow velocities exceed the Nyquist limit aliasing occurs, as can be seen i.e. in Fig. 6.89 (p. 110) and 6.92 (p. 111). Typically, turbulence is observed in conditions of jet-like streaming as found in stenoses, regurgitations or high-pressure shunts. These turbulent jets are surrounded by eddies and vortices which may be imaged by a multicolored *mosaic*-like imaging pattern (see Figs. 6.70, p. 99,

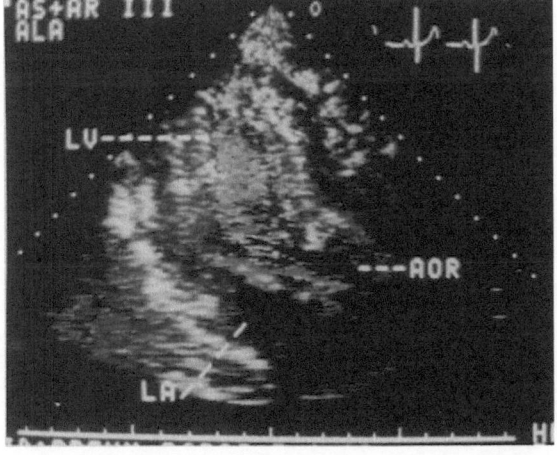

Fig. 4.5 Motions of the cardiac walls and valves in severe aortic incompetence. Apical long axis view of the left ventricle *(LV)* (RBG2). Early diastolic frame. The left ventricular cavity is expanding, thereby causing the anterior and posterior wall of the ventricle to move away from the transducer which causes them to appear *blue*. At the same time the anterior leaflet of the mitral valve is starting to open with a movement towards the transducer and is therefore colored *red*. In contrast to the clear colors of the walls and the mitral valve indicating identical Doppler shift for the cardiac structures. The regurgitant blood in the left ventricle appears a more mixed color (see text). The jet splashes directly into the LV cavity without touching the mitral valve or the septum

6.101, p. 116). It is not always possible to differentiate between aliasing caused by high velocities of the jet or by vortex formation. However, the appearance of a mosaic pattern is always considered to be pathognomonic for abnormal flow conditions and is found in stenoses, regurgitations, or shunts.

4.7 Differentiation of Flow Velocities from Wall Motion

A differentiation of flow velocities from the motion of walls or valves is usually possible because of the difference in their Doppler frequency spectrum. Blood cells as ultrasound reflectors of the streaming blood move with similar but not completely identical velocities. In comparison, the motion of walls and of valves is completely uniform. Therefore the moving structures are characterized by virtually no variance in color display whereas blood flow is imaged with much more variance (Fig. 4.5). It is important to realize this because in jet-like flow conditions, the activation of the display function of tissue priority may suppress the origin of the jet (see section 3.3 and Fig. 3.6, p. 18).

5 Physiological Flow Velocity Patterns in the Cardiovascular System

This chapter will describe the distribution of blood flow velocities under physiological conditions and in secondary functional disturbances within the heart and the great vessels. The spatial as well as the temporal distribution for every compartment will yield a topography of flow behavior in the cardiovascular system. The directions in normal as well as in pathological states, however, do not always obey the rules for the standardization of echocardiographic views as proposed by the American Society of Echocardiography in 1980 [20]. Thus, in many cases it is necessary to change the orientation of the sector plane from the usual image orientations in order to cover the area of flow extension as far as possible. This may sometimes render the anatomical interpretation of the resulting images difficult at first glance.

5.1 Left Atrium and Pulmonary Veins

In most patients flow velocities in the left atrium are not high enough to be imaged all over the left atrial cavity. It is only displayed in its infero-distal part proximal to the mitral valve (see Fig. 2.1, p.7, Figs. 5.5a+b, p.30) where convective acceleration towards the mitral orifice takes place.

In high-flow states, such as considerable left-to-right shunts, the inflow of the pulmonary veins (Fig. 5.1) or the whole cavity of the two atria (Fig. 5.2) may be visualized. This occurs mainly during the ejection time in systole and for most of the diastole until atrial contraction (Fig. 5.3). Just before atrial contraction and during the isovolumetric contraction phase of ventricular systole, flow velocities in the left atrium are low.

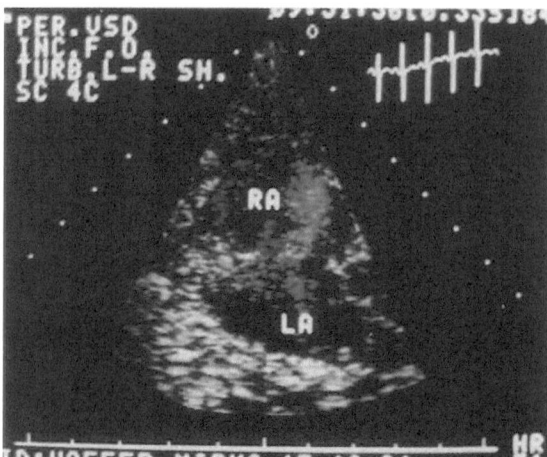

Fig. 5.1 Visualization of pulmonary venous flow within the left atrium in ventricular septal defect *(VSD)* and incomplete foramen ovale. Subcostal four-chamber view (RB2). Blood from the lower pulmonary veins of both sides is seen to drain into the left atrium *(LA)* from where a left-to-right shunt crosses the atrial septum into the right atrium *(RA)*. The ventricles are positioned on the right side of the image

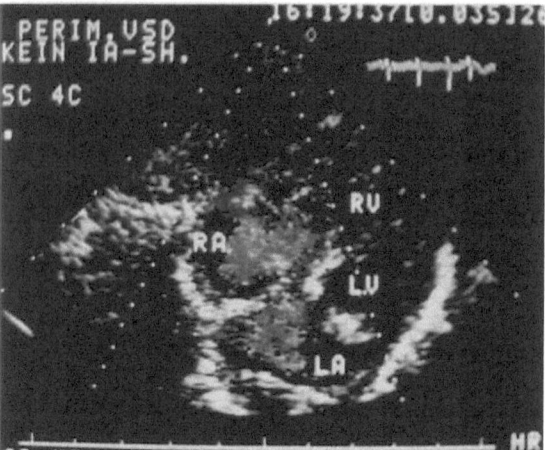

Fig. 5.2 Blood flow display in both atria in a state of high cardiac output. Subcostal four-chamber view (RBG2). Both atria show equal intensity and distribution of flow velocities, there is no shunt

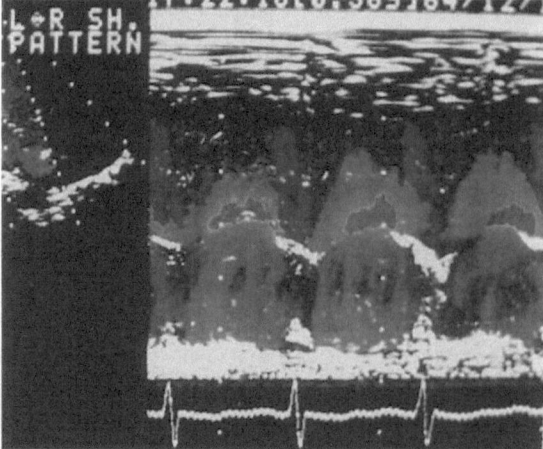

Fig. 5.3 Time distribution of pulmonary venous blood flow in the left atrium in ventricular septal defect *(VSD)* with considerable left-to-right shunt and incomplete foramen ovale (RB2). Flow ceases during atrial contraction and isovolumetric contraction of the ventricles. Interatrial left-to-right shunt shows alias. See text for more details

5.2 Mitral Valve

The function of the mitral valve is to connect the left atrium to the left ventricle in diastole and to separate both chambers in systole. CBFI demonstrates that between the two phases of diastolic inflow there may be a short episode of "diastolic mitral regurgitation," as can be seen in Figure 5.4a.

During systole the mitral valve is closed and directs the outflowing blood from the left ventricle into the aortic root (blue area in Fig. 5.4). In the M/Q-mode the closure line of the mitral valve remains free of color, indicating systolic competence of the valve. It can be seen from Fig. 5.4b that the color display corresponds exactly to the FFT spectral analysis in respect to flow direction and timing.

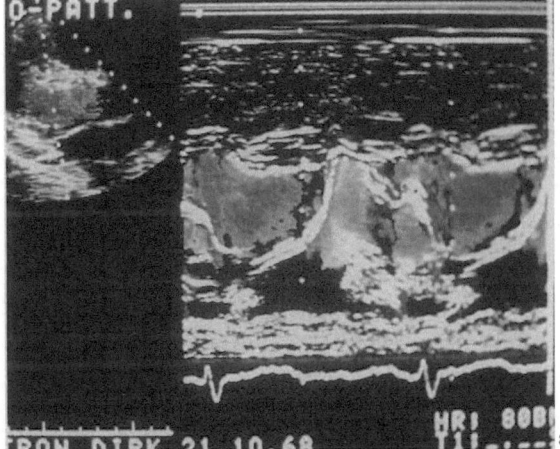

Fig. 5.4a, b Normal time sequence of mitral blood flow velocities, RBG2. The biphasic filling pattern of the left ventricle is clearly visible. In late diastole, immediately before the atrial filling period, a short phase of "diastolic regurgitation" can be seen. The left ventricular outflow is filled with blood flowing towards the aortic root, this flow movement is continued uninterruptedly into systole.
a M/Q-mode with 2D color insert

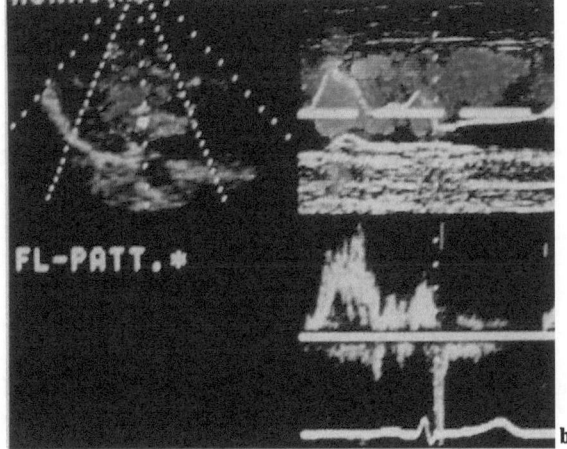

b M/Q-mode and FFT single gate trace together with 2D color insert. The position of the sample volume is indicated by the *interrupted line* in the M/Q-mode and by the *dot* in the 2D colour insert. See text for more details

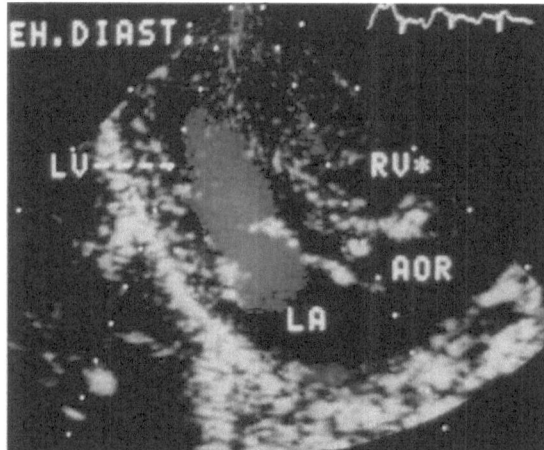

Fig. 5.5a-c Spatial distribution of flow vectors in the left ventricular inflow tract, at different points in time and in different views; it is relatively flat under normal conditions.
a Early diastolic inflow, apical long axis view (RB2)

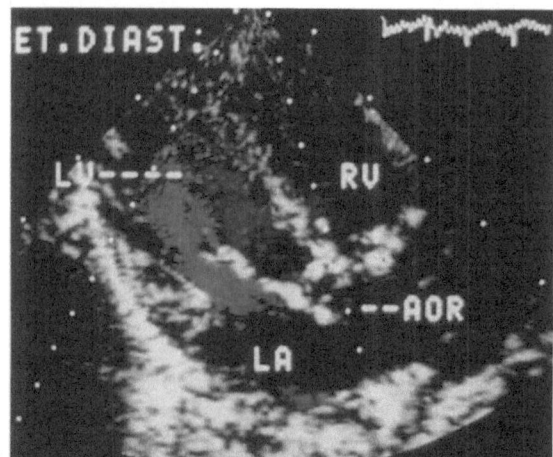

b Late diastolic inflow, same position and color settings as **a**. Blood is seen to flow around the tip of the anterior mitral leaflet thereby filling the left ventricular outflow *(blue)*

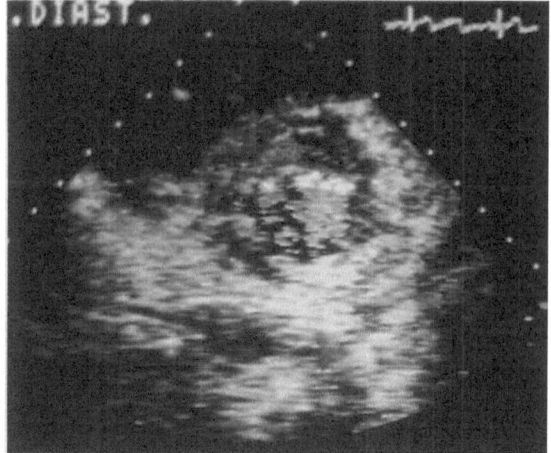

c Early diastolic inflow, parasternal short axis view (RBG2). Inflow is imaged in *orange-yellow*, diastolic filling of the outflow tract is imaged in *blue. AOR,* aortic root

Under normal conditions the flow profile across the mitral orifice is relatively flat (Fig. 5.5) but in high-flow states like post-tricuspid left-to-right shunts or anemia there is an uneven distribution of flow vectors with higher velocities towards the anterior mitral valve leaflet and the interventricular septum. The sectional area of the mitral orifice is normally filled almost completely by velocities of the inflowing blood (Fig. 5.5 c).

5.3 Left Ventricle

The left ventricle represents the pumping chamber for the systemic circulation. It receives the blood from the left atrium through the mitral valve in diastole and pumps it into the aorta in systole. This is shown in Fig. 2.1, p. 7. Flow topography of the left ventricle is relatively complex because there is no separation of inflow and outflow tract. With advancing diastole, blood flow in the left ventricular cavity changes its direction and flows around the anterior mitral leaflet into the left ventricular outflow tract (Fig. 5.5 b, c). This flow movement is continued without interruption into systole and stops with the beginning of isovolumetric relaxation of the left ventricle (Fig. 5.4). The flow profile in the left ventricular outflow tract is variable, as in the right ventricle: on one hand it may be found to be relatively flat, on the other, it may be skewed (see Figs. 2.4a, p. 9 and 2.5b, p. 10).

5.4 Aorta (Ascending, Arch, Descending)

The aorta receives the blood ejected from the left ventricle. Normally the aortic valve opens completely, aligning the leaflets parallel to the blood stream (Figs. 5.6 and 5.7). The *aortic root* is, however, not uniformly filled by the streaming blood. Between the aortic leaflets and the wall, in Valsalva's sinuses, there are special flow conditions. Blood flows backwards into each of the three sinuses around the free edges of the leaflets (Fig. 5.8). This may help to keep the valve in a position ready to close as soon as the left ventricular pressure falls below the aortic pressure with virtually no regurgitation. In diastole there is no significant blood flow velocity in the aortic root so the leaflets remain colorless.

In the *ascending aorta* the systolic flow profile is usually not flat, as stated by other authors [25]. Sometimes we found the velocity to be higher in the postero-lateral parts than in the antero-medial parts, as described by Jenni et al. [25], in other healthy individuals blood flow velocity is highest in the central part of the ascending aorta (see Fig. 5.10). In diastole no significant flow velocities are visualized. The *aortic arch* and *descending aorta*

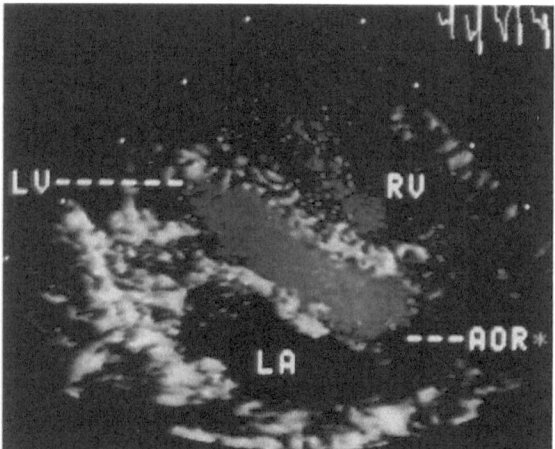

Fig. 5.6 Normal left ventricular outflow tract and aortic root *(AOR)*. Parasternal long axis view, systolic frame. The leaflets of the aortic valve are seen to open widely aligning themselves parallel to the aortic wall to give way to the outflowing blood. Convective acceleration along the outflow tract into the aortic root is recognizable by a gradual increase in color brightness (RB2). Additionally it is evident that blood is flowing faster near the interventricular septum than at the posterior wall of the outflow and the aortic root

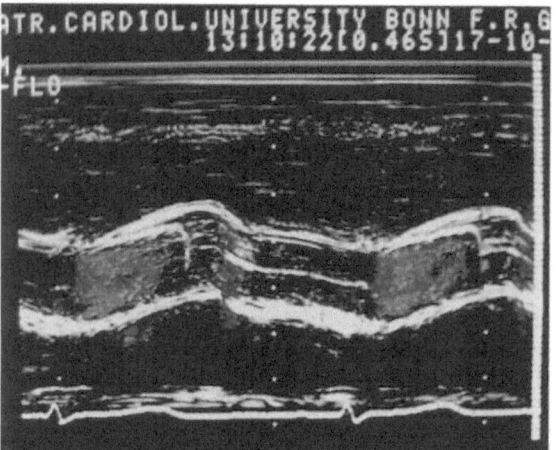

Fig. 5.7 Normal flow through the aortic valve, M/Q-mode (RBG2). The typical systolic opening box of the aortic leaflets is filled by blue-encoded blood flow. Decreasing color brightness during systole signifies the regression of flow velocity which is more pronounced near the posterior wall. In the last part of systole velocity values are below the display threshold before the valve closes and causes coloration of the closing line

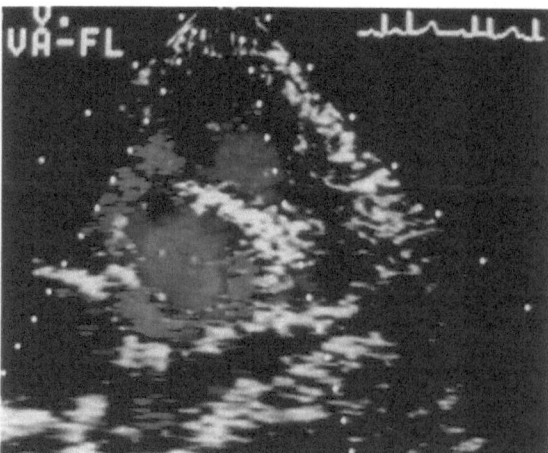

Fig. 5.8 Normal flow in the aortic root, parasternal short axis view (RB2). Maximal velocity 46 cm/s. Flow within the valve orifice is imaged in *blue* as away-flow; in Valsalva's sinuses between the free edges of the cusps and the wall, there is towards-flow *(red)*. See text fore more details

Fig. 5.9a, b Normal flow velocity profile in the distal aortic arch (**a**) and the descending aorta (**b**).
a Distal aortic arch, suprasternal position (RB1). A symmetrically parabolic profile is visualized by the central aliasing to *red* along the aortic lumen. *VCS*, superior caval vein

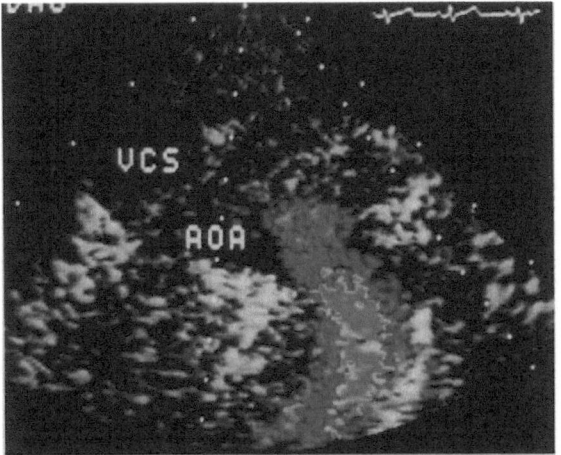

b Descending aorta (*DAO*), subcostal position (RB2). The flow profile is similar to that found in the distal aortic arch as can be judged from the central aliasing to *blue*

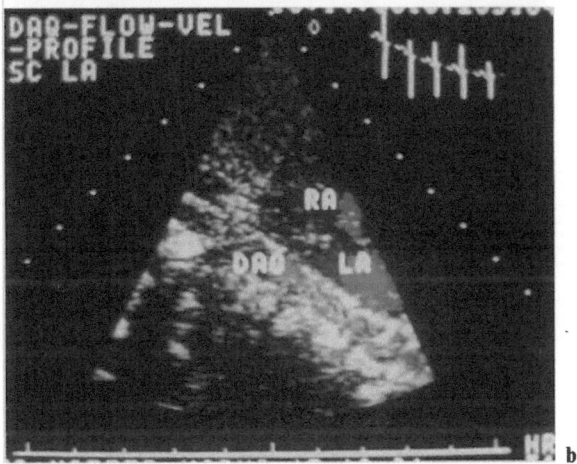

have a similar flow pattern, except that at the beginning of the descending aorta there is a typical parabolic flow profile (Fig. 5.9a + b). Significantly, flow velocities occur only in systole (see Fig. 6.67, p. 97).

5.5 Right Atrium and Caval Veins

Most of the systemic venous blood reaches the *right atrium* via both caval veins, only a small amount is normally contributed by the coronary sinus. The superior vena cava (VCS) can be visualized from the suprasternal position chosing a sector plane which cuts the aortic arch almost transversally. Figure 5.10a shows the VCS, which is normally on the right side, in a longitudinal section. Figure 5.10b shows a left-sided VCS. Blood is flow-

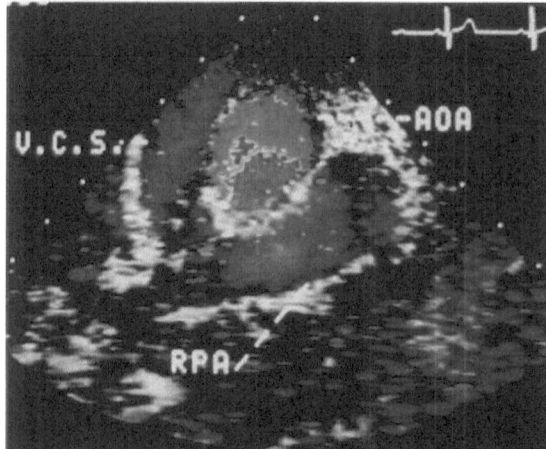

a

Fig. 5.10 a, b Blood flow in the superior caval vein *(VCS)*. Suprasternal long axis view of VCS (RB2). Away-flow towards the right atrium is imaged in *blue*.
a Normally, the VCS runs on the right side. In the aortic arch *(AOA)* the higher velocities at the inferior medial wall are causing aliasing *(blue)* whereas the lower velocities at the superior lateral wall are displayed in the original color. *RPA*, right pulmonic artery branch

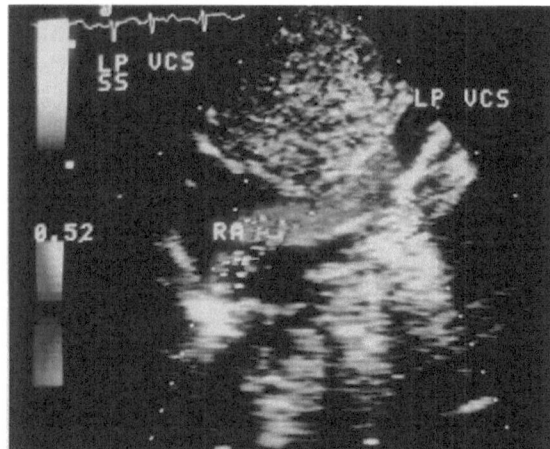

b

b Sometimes, a persistent left VCS is found which may drain to the coronary sinus from the left side *(LP VCS)*

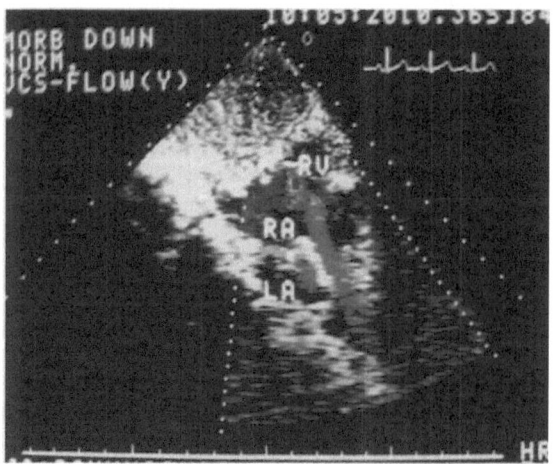

Fig. 5.11 Emptying of the VCS into the right atrium viewed from the subcostal position in the short axis (RB2). See text for more details

Fig. 5.12 Flow velocities in the inferior caval vein and the hepatic veins in an individual after successful surgical correction of tetralogy of Fallot (RB1). For most of the cardiac cycle blood is flowing away *(blue)* towards the right atrium (T1), after artial contraction (T2) towards flow (red) can be seen because of decrease in contractility of the right ventricle. Short periods of towards-flow may, however, be observed also in normal individuals (see text)

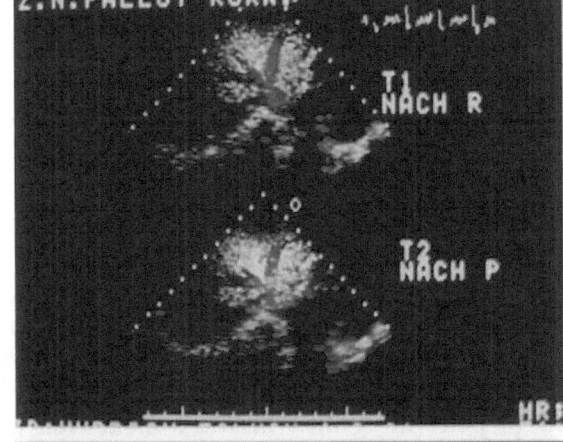

Fig. 5.13a, b Flow patterns in hepatic veins and interior vena cava. **a** Physiological flow pattern in a hepatic vein which corresponds to the flow in the inferior vena cava (RBG2). The typical four-phasic flow pattern which corresponds to the well-known pressure trace is easily recognizable in the M/Q-mode and the FFT trace

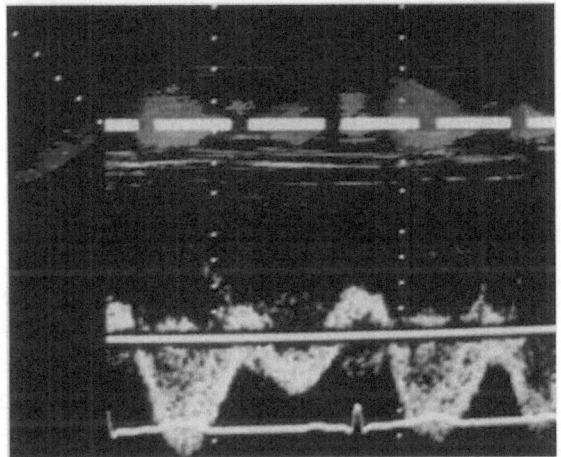

a

b M/Q-mode showing a wave-dependent backflow *(red)* into the inferior caval vein (VCI) (RB1)

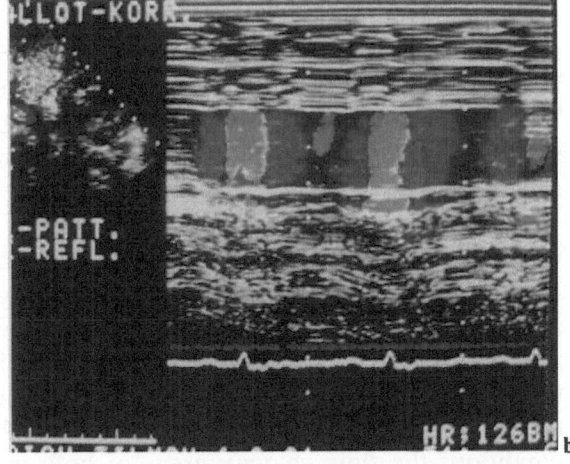

b

ing away from the transducer. The emptying of the VCS into the right atrium can also be visualized in the subcostal short axis view (Fig. 5.11). Blood flows towards the transducer through the right atrium and is directed towards the tricuspid orifice. In the middle of the atrial cavity it crosses the blood stream of the inferior vena cava (VCI), which is directed towards the interatrial septum (blue in Fig. 5.11).

The VCI is best visualized from the subcostal position in a long axis plane. Additionally, some hepatic veins can be visualized. In Fig. 5.12 the drainage of the VCI into the right atrium can be seen, normally there is away-flow (upper picture T1 in Fig. 5.12). The physiological flow pattern of the VCI is shown in Fig. 5.13 a. To obtain a better angle between flow vector and ultrasound beam the flow trace was recorded in one hepatic vein where the flow pattern is identical to that in the caval vein. In coughing or performing the Valsalva's maneuver, however, backflow from the right atrium may be observed (lower picture T2 in Fig. 5.12). This also occurs in pathological conditions such as in severe tricuspid regurgitation (see p. 107), in an atrial septal defect at the end of systole and the beginning of diastole, and in heavily increased right ventricular afterload during atrial contraction (Fig. 5.13).

5.6 Tricuspid Valve

The tricuspid valve serves the same purpose as the mitral valve. In several respects, however, the blood flow behavior is different. Under normal conditions we have never observed a so-called diastolic tricuspid regurgitation like that of the mitral valve, despite the fact that transtricuspid flow is biphasic too (Fig. 5.14). The explanation may be that the right ventricle is much more compliant than the left because of the much lower myocardial mass and therefore does not reflect the diastolic filling wave. In most normal individuals there is a small amount of tricuspid regurgitation which has also been observed by other investigators [67]. A typical finding of this "physiological" incompetence is that it may be of short duration during systole (Fig. 5.14b) and that the extension in the right atrium is small (Fig. 5.15).

Under normal flow conditions the velocity profile across the tricuspid orifice is flat (Fig. 5.14a), but transition to a parabolic profile may occur in high-flow states, i. e., in pretricuspid left-to-right shunts (Fig. 5.16b). This may cause a "functional" tricuspid stenosis because of a high volume flow rate. In Fig. 5.16b it can also be seen that in this condition the flow velocity area of the tricuspid valve is much larger and is much brighter than that of the mitral valve and there is additional aliasing. Under normal flow conditions the flow velocity areas of both atrioventricular valves are of similar size and color brightness (Fig. 5.16a).

Fig. 5.14a, b Normal diastolic inflow into the right ventricle *(RV)* via the tricuspid valve, parasternal short axis view (RBG2).
a The whole right ventricle *(RV)*, including the outflow tract and the main pulmonary artery, is visualized, flow can only be seen at the tricuspid valve. The flow profile is flat

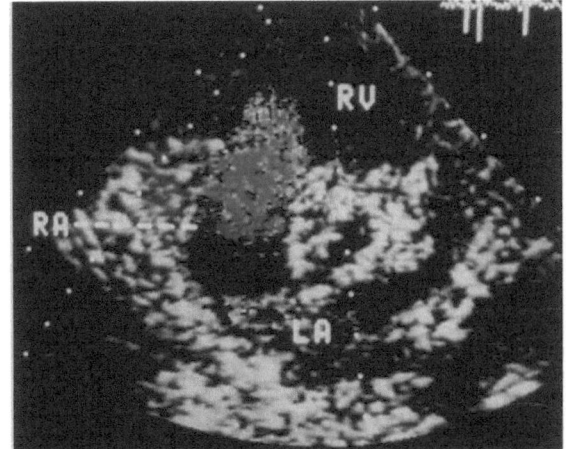

b M/Q-mode showing a normal flow pattern across the tricuspid valve (RBG2). In diastole this is biphasic, there is a systolic backflow of short duration into the right atrium (turquoise, marked by three asterisks) which represents a "physiological" tricuspid regurgitation

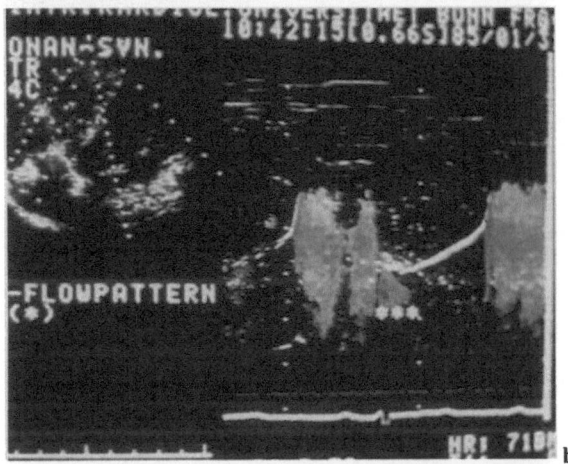

Fig. 5.15 "Physiological" tricuspid regurgitation, apical four-chamber view (RBG2). In this early systolic frame a small amount of regurgitation into the right atrium *(turquoise)* can be seen, while the mitral valve does not exhibit any leakage

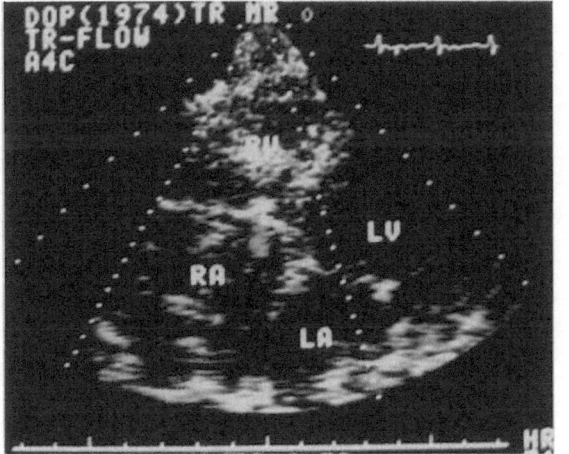

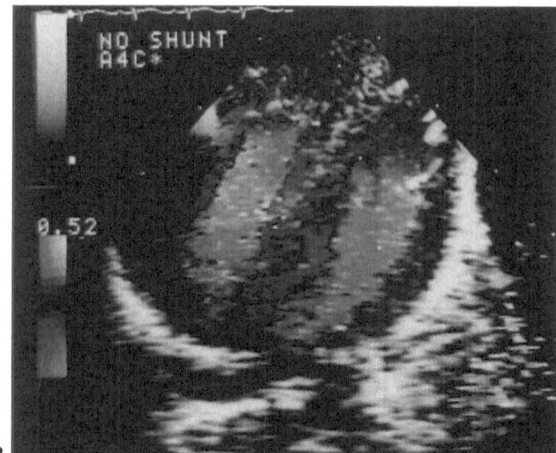

a

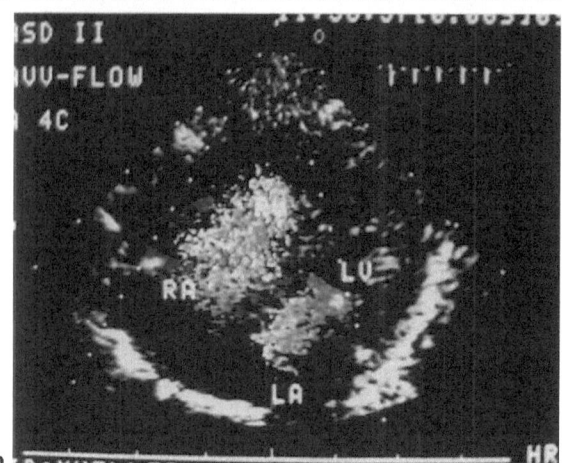

b

Fig.5.16a, b Early diastolic flow through both atrioventricular valves, apical four-chamber view (RBG2).
a Normal individual. Brightness and extension of the ventricular inflow areas are similar, the walls of the chambers are colored *blue* because of their expansion towards the cardiac base

b Pretricuspid left-to-right shunt causes tricuspid volume load which is visualized by *brighter colors* together with some aliasing and a greater flow area across the tricuspid valve

5.7 Right Ventricle

The right ventricle serves as the pumping chamber for the pulmonary circulation. Inflow and outflow tracts are clearly separated and cannot be completely visualized together in one plane. Because of this spatial separation, blood flow velocities have slowed down considerably as the diastolic filling wave reaches the distal part of the outflow tract (Fig.5.14a). In systole the flow profile in the outflow tract is not always flat as proposed by other authors [56], but may become markedly parabolic in high-flow states, i.e., in left-to-right shunts (Fig.5.17).

Fig. 5.17 Flow profile in the right ventricular outflow *(RVO)* and main pulmonary artery *(MPA)* in ventricular septal defect *(VSD)* with moderate left-to-right shunt volume. Parasternal long axis view of RVO (RB1). Systolic frame. A typical parabolic flow profile has built up reaching from the RVO far into the MPA

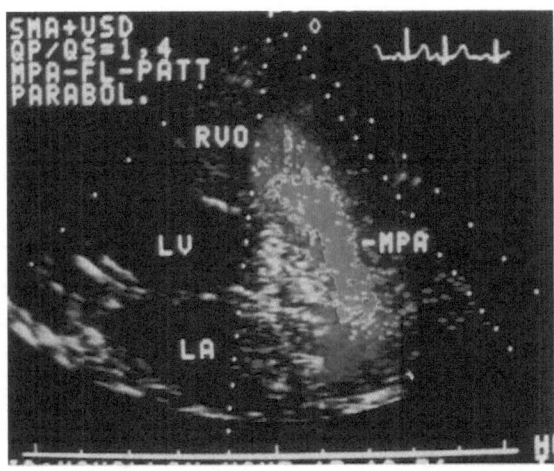

5.8 Pulmonary Artery and Main Branches

The MPA receives blood from the right ventricle and takes it to the lung. The pulmonic valve opens completely but in contrast to the aortic root we have not observed a space with different flow velocity distribution between the leaflets and the wall (see Fig. 5.20b). With the onset of diastole there is pronounced backflow of short duration towards the pulmonic orifice (Fig. 5.18). This may help to close the pulmonic valve and is in contrast to the flow patterns in the aortic root where we have not observed such backflow velocities. Pulmonary regurgitation is commonly seen in

Fig. 5.18 M/Q-mode of pulmonary artery flow in a normsl subject (RBG2). Systolic flow is coded in *blue* as away-flow, in early diastole there is a short episode of backflow towards the pulmonary valve *(orange)* which is normal and may help to close the pulmonic valve

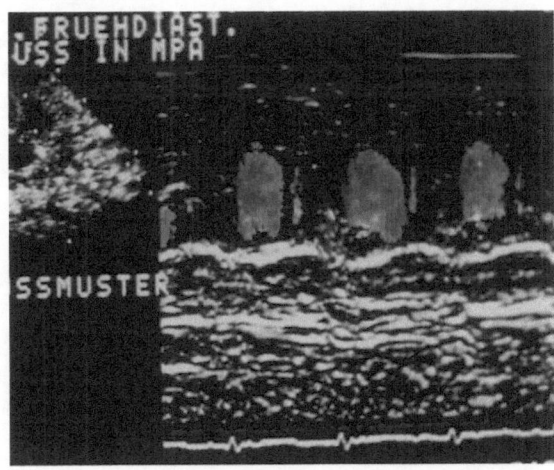

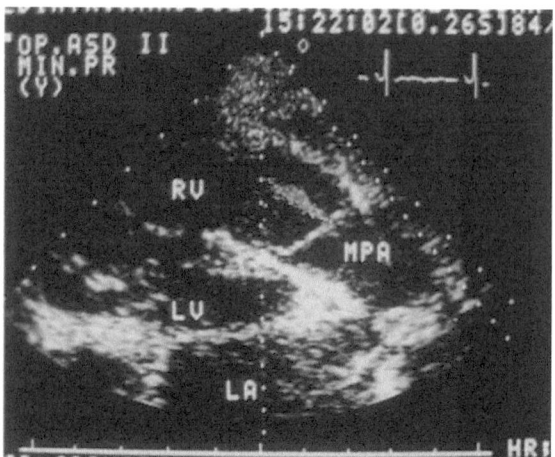

Fig. 5.19 Slight pulmonary regurgitation, parasternal long axis view of main pulmonary artery *(MPA)* in late diastole. The *orange-yellow jet* represents a small amount of regurgitant blood. This is often seen in normal subjects

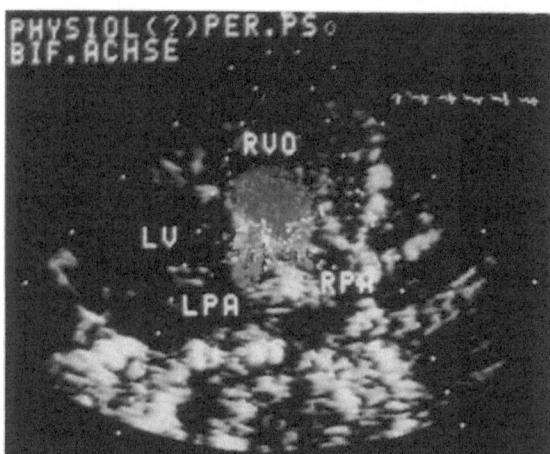

Fig. 5.20 a, b Systolic flow in the main pulmonary artery *(MPA)* and the proximal part of its two branches. Parasternal short axis view of the base (RBG2).
a In neonates vortex formation at the bifurcation in common because of slight peripheral stenoses which are physiological for this age

a

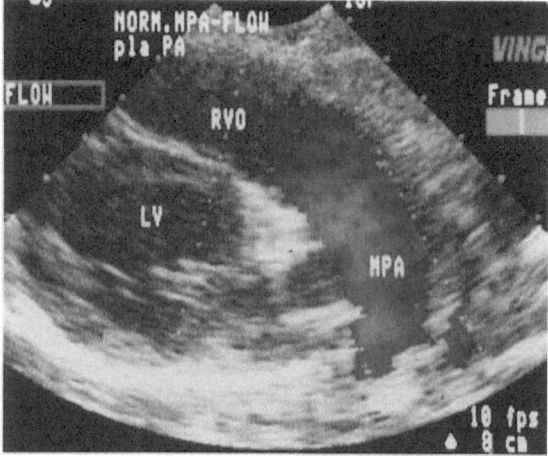

b Later in life blood flows undisturbed from the MPA into both branches

b

healthy individuals and may be the consequence of this valve closure mechanism (Fig. 5.19).

The a-dip in the M-mode trace of pulmonic valve motion has been the subject of ample speculations. Feigenbaum [14, p. 391] has suggested that it may represent an opening motion of the valve caused by the atrial contribution to diastolic filling which leads to outflow into the MPA. Figure 2.3 b (p. 8) shows no color in late diastole which could indicate considerable blood flow into the pulmonary artery. This reflects our experience, which indicates that the a-wave may not reflect outflow of the right ventricle.

Blood flow profile in the MPA is virtually never flat. In a recently published study [53], we found in 48 of 50 individuals parabolic flow profile with longitudinal acceleration leading to considerably higher velocities in the central part of MPA than at the edges or in the proximal and distal parts. This makes the reliability of single gate Doppler measurements of cardiac output in the pulmonary artery with arbitrary positioning of the sample volume questionable.

The MPA divides into two branches which can be visualized from the parasternal position in many patients (Fig. 5.20). In neonates the occurrence of vortices at the bifurcation is common (Fig. 5.20 a) and may be caused by "physiological" peripheral stenoses which have been described by Rudolph [59].

6 Blood Flow Velocity Patterns in Heart Disease

Flow patterns in heart disease are changed in one or more respects compared to *normal* flow: characteristics of the normal flow are that it occurs at the right place at the right time with normal velocities (right in space, right in time, right in velocity). Pathological flow patterns in heart disease may exhibit pathological characteristics, such as turbulence and vortex formation, or they may occur at the wrong time or at the wrong location.

6.1 Shunts at or Above Atrial Level (Pretricuspid Shunts)

Shunts at or above atrial level can be grouped together as pretricuspid shunt lesions. They have in common the fact that they take place in the low-pressure part of the circulation and that they lead to volume load of the tricuspid valve and the right ventricle. Only rarely is the flow velocity high enough to cause disturbed flow and the formation of vortices in the shunt area. This is therefore an example of flow with normal velocities occurring at the wrong place and is therefore termed "pathological."

6.1.1 Incomplete Foramen Ovale. An incomplete foramen ovale is, in our experience, a common finding in healthy neonates. Its characteristic finding is a left-to-right shunt at atrial level without a visible defect of the atrial septum. The shunt is much more pronounced and shows higher velocities in coexisting heart disease with left ventricular volume or pressure load (see Figure 5.3, p. 28). In contrast to a secundum atrial septal defect, there is no detectable right-to-left shunt. The interatrial shunt disappears in the first few months of life despite the fact that the foramen ovale may be still patent.

6.1.2 Secundum Atrial Septal Defect. An atrial septal defect is most commonly found in the position of the embryological *ostium secundum* (ASD II) which corresponds to the area of the foramen ovale. The defect is easily detected by 2D echocardiography [4, 64]. Fig. 6.1 a shows a small ASD II in the subcostal four-chamber view. CBFI helps to visualize the

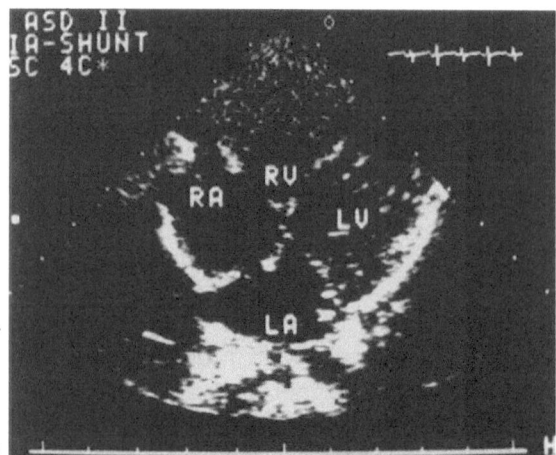

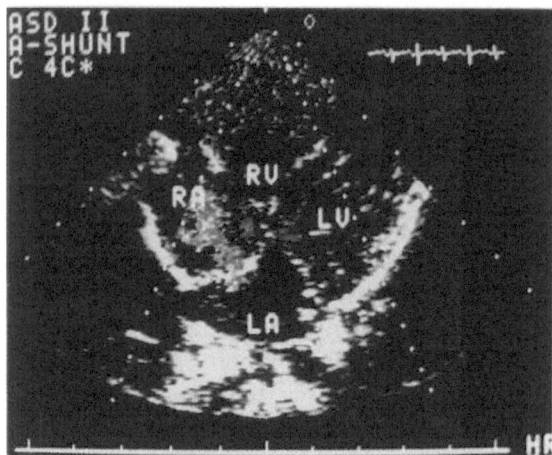

Fig. 6.1 a, b Small atrial septal defect of secundum type (ASD II) from the subcostal position.
a The 2D echocardiogram shows an echo drop-out of the interatrial septum with increased ultrasound reflectance from the margin of the basal part of the septum

b When CBFI is added (RBG2), the interatrial left-to-right shunt in early systole is visualized as towards-flow in *orange-yellow* and occupies a smaller area in the right atrium *(RA)* than a large ASD II, as shown in Fig. 6.2

left-to-right shunt across the atrial septum (Fig. 6.1 b). Larger defects show a larger area in the right atrium occupied by blood cells with the typical left-to-right shunt velocities (Fig. 6.2) than smaller defects. The echocardiographically determined defect diameter does not correlate well with the amount of left-to-right shunt [15] but there is evidence that the size of the shunt-flow-velocity area shows a better correlation [31, 32].

A special diagnostic value of CBFI lies in the detection of left-to-right shunts across fenestrated defects which cannot be diagnosed by 2D echocardiography alone [15]. Figure 6.3 shows the left-to-right shunt across a fenestrated ASD II with moderate amount of left-to-right shunt volume. The 2D image (Fig. 6.3 a) shows two drop-outs which may or may not be defects but convincing evidence comes from the display by CBFI (Fig. 6.3 b).

Uncomplicated ASDs exhibit a typical bidirectional shunt pattern [26, 52]. Left-to-right shunting takes the most time during the cardiac cycle

Fig. 6.2 Large secundum atrial septal defect. Subcostal position, late diastole. CBFI visualizes the left-to-right shunt across a large ASD II which occupies a larger area in the RA than that in Fig. 6.1 b

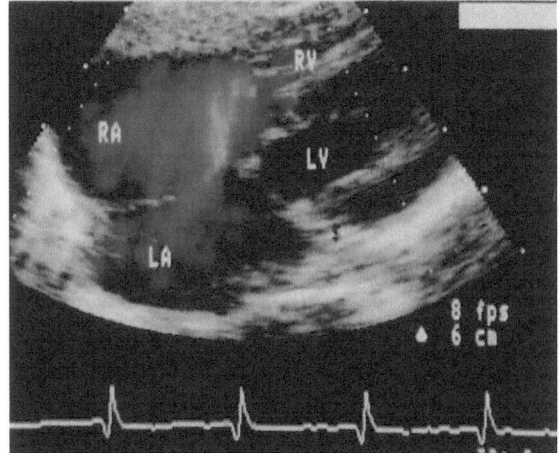

Fig. 6.3 a, b A fenestrated secundum atrial septal defect *(ASD II)* from the subcostal position in mid-systole.
a The 2D echocardiogram shows two interruptions of the atrial septum and two small echo reflections in the right atrium *(A)* which may be caused by parts of the dislocated flap of the foramen ovale

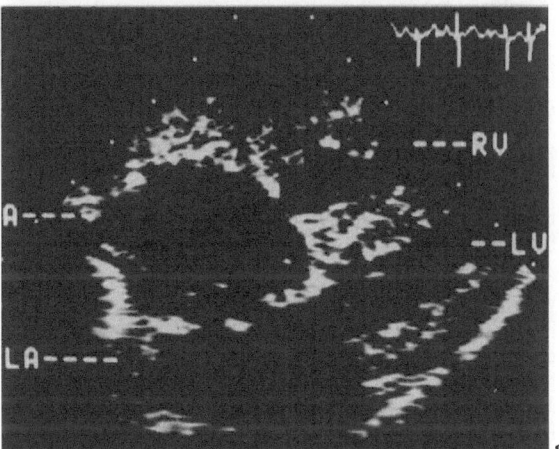

b CBFI (RBG2) shows left-to-right shunt through two separate defects in secundum position and the deflectance of shunt flow towards the tricuspid valve by rudimentary parts of the flap of the foramen ovale

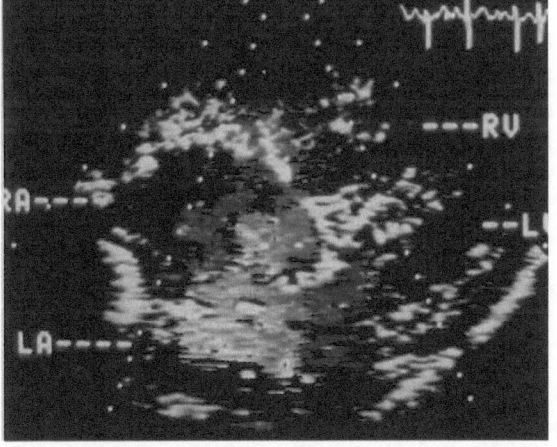

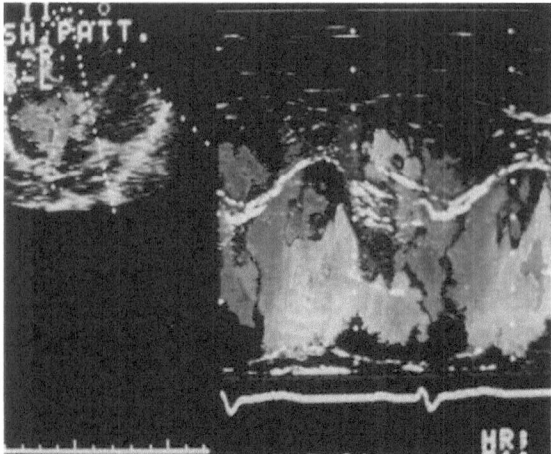

Fig. 6.4 Time distribution of interatrial shunting in uncomplicated secundum atrial septal defects *(ASD II)*. M/Q-mode (RBG2) demonstrates the interatrial shunt pattern. The *undulating line* above the shunt flow represents the tricuspid valve ring. During most of the cardiac cycle there is left-to-right shunt with maximal velocity at the end of systole and the beginning of diastole, as can be seen from color aliasing near the tricuspid valve ring. There is, however, also a short period of right-to-left shunt *(blue vertical flow area)* which takes place at the beginning of systole and seems to be caused by systolic closure of the tricuspid valve and the concomitant tricuspid regurgitation which starts at the tricuspid valve

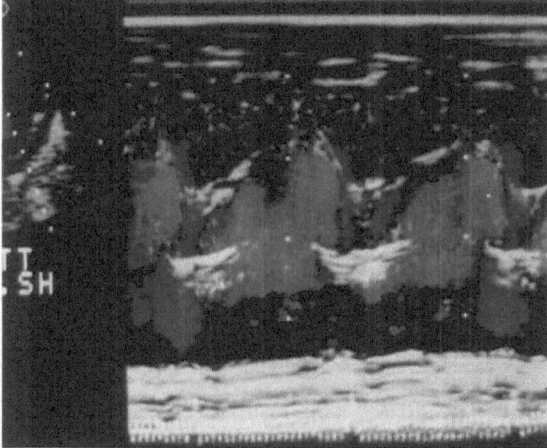

Fig. 6.5 Interatrial *(IA)* shunt pattern in secundum atrial septal defect complicated by concomitant heart disease. Interatrial shunt pattern in pulmonic stenosis with right ventricular hypertrophy (RB2). Prominent right-to left (1st and 3rd cardiac cycle) shunt is caused by the decrease in right ventricular compliance and takes place in late diastole (blue)

(red-yellow in Fig. 6.4) but invariably there is also a short interval of right-to-left shunting occurring during the isovolumetric contraction phase in early systole (blue in Fig. 6.4). The right-to-left shunt seems to be initiated by the systolic closure of the tricuspid valve (Fig. 6.4a) and is found to change with deep respiration. In complicated defects with a decrease in right ventricular compliance, the right-to-left shunt component becomes more pronounced by taking more time of the cardiac cycle and occupying more space in the left atrium (Fig. 6.5). If the defect is complicated by heart disease causing a decrease in left ventricular compliance, for instance in left ventricular outflow tract stenosis, cardiomyopathy, in posttricuspid left-to-right shunts, or in left ventricular inflow tract stenosis (i.e., Lutembacher's syndrome) the interatrial left-to-right shunt velocity increases hereby causing aliasing and reducing or eliminating the right-to-left shunt component (see Fig. 5.3, p. 28).

In *conclusion,* the interatrial shunt pattern in ASD is modified by accompanying heart disease, the cause of which may be a decrease in compliance of the right or left ventricle.

6.1.3 Primum Atrial Septal Defect. Atrial septal defects of the ostium primum type (ASD I) are caused by the nonexistance of the embryological ostium primum which forms the caudal part of the interatrial septum immediately above the atrioventricular valve level. It is commonly accompanied by atrioventricular valve clefts, especially of the mitral valve, and by ventricular septal defects of the atrioventricular type as part of the so-called endocardial cushion defect. Figure 6.6a shows an ASD I which is typically positioned immediately above the atrioventricular valve level; Fig. 6.6b shows the left-to-right shunt across the defect in early diastole into the right atrium as blood begins to enter the right ventricle. The

Fig. 6.6a–c Atrial septal defect of the ostium primum type *(ASD I)*. Apical four-chamber view.
a The 2D echocardiogram shows an echo drop-out of the interatrial septum immediately above the atrioventricular valve level.

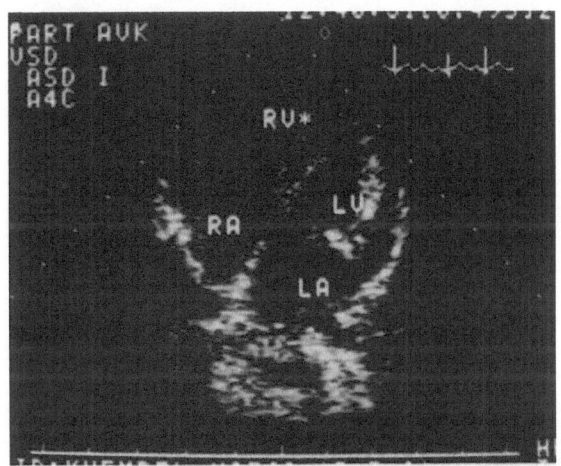

b Left-to-right shunt (RBG2) becomes visible as CBFI is added to the 2D image.

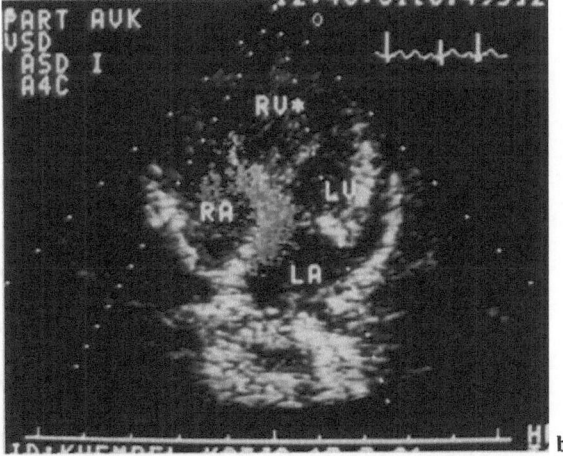

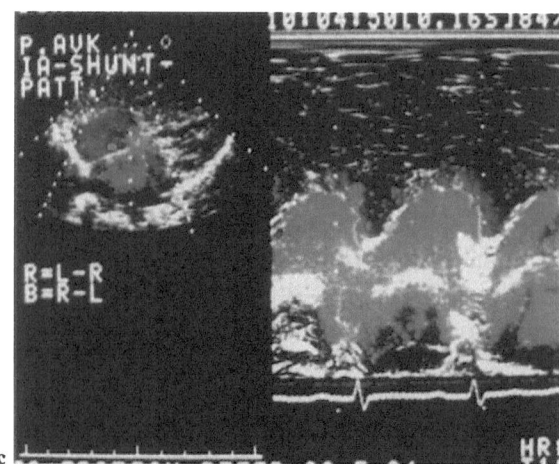

c M/Q-mode showing the time distribution of the shunt flow in another defect of the septum primum (RB2). There is a continuous left-to-right shunt without any episode of right-to-left shunt

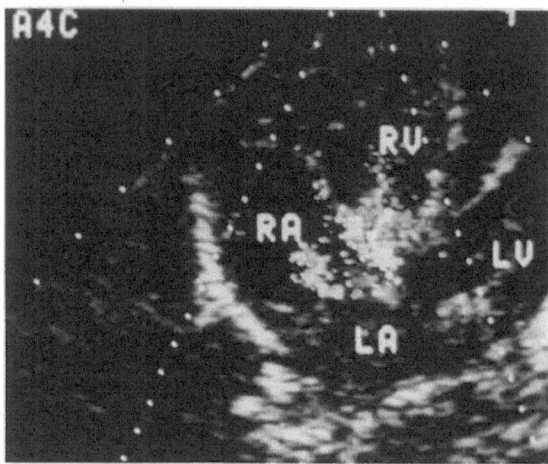

Fig. 6.7 Left-to-right shunt across two coexisting atrial defects. Apical four-chamber view (RBG1). Systolic frame. The shunt through the ASD II is visualized in a more cephalad position whereas the ASD I is found in the typical location above the atrioventricular valves. Additionally there is a small degree of tricuspid incompetence *(turquoise)*. To show the flow velocities more clearly, the RBG1 display mode has been chosen.

time course of the shunt is different from that seen in ASD II (see p. 45), a consistent right-to-left direction of the shunt is frequently missing (Fig. 6.6c).

In *complete endocardial cushion defects* the shunt pattern may change due to additionally existing cardiac defects (see p. 67). Sometimes it may be combined with an ASD II as is demonstrated in Fig. 6.7. In this special case CBFI was the only method by which the coexistence of the two interatrial shunts could be diagnosed preoperatively.

6.1.4 Sinus Venosus Atrial Septal Defect. ASDs of the sinus venosus type are positioned in the cranial part of the interatrial septum near the orifice of the VCS and usually combined with an anomalous return of the right-sided pulmonary veins into the right atrium. Their echocardiographic visu-

Fig. 6.8a-c Pretricuspid left-to-right shunts other than ASD II or ASD I.

a Left-to-right shunt across a sinus venosus atrial septal defect visualized in the subcostal short axis view (RBG2). Early diastole. The shunt flow is detectable only in this position together with the anomalous drainage of the right pulmonary veins

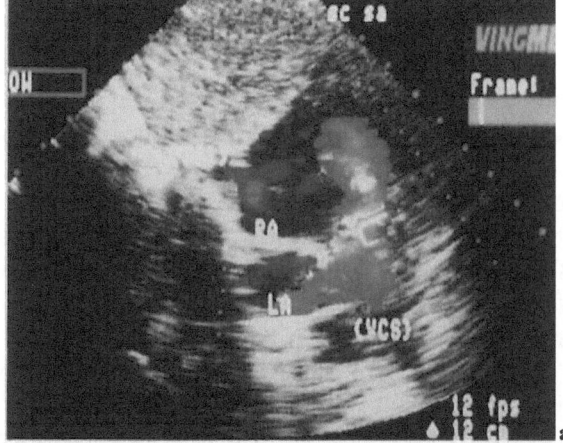

b Partial anomalous pulmonary venous drainage into the superior caval vein *(VCS)* leads to an increase in venous backflow into the right atrium *(RA)* and is viewed in the subcostal short axis view (RBG2)

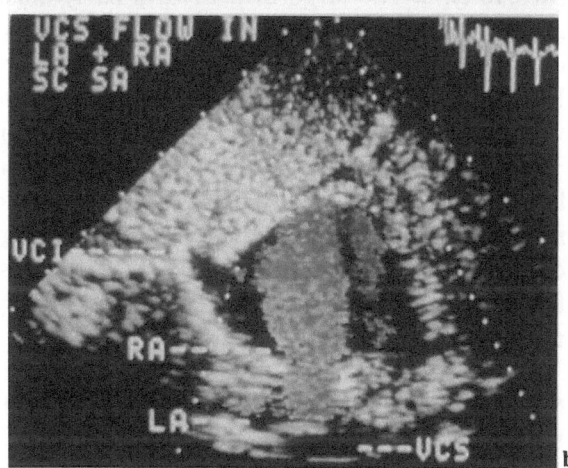

c Total anomalous pulmonary venous drainage into the portal vein *(asterisk)*, visualized in a subcostal long axis view of the portal vein. Turbulence is a sign of stenosis at the drainage site

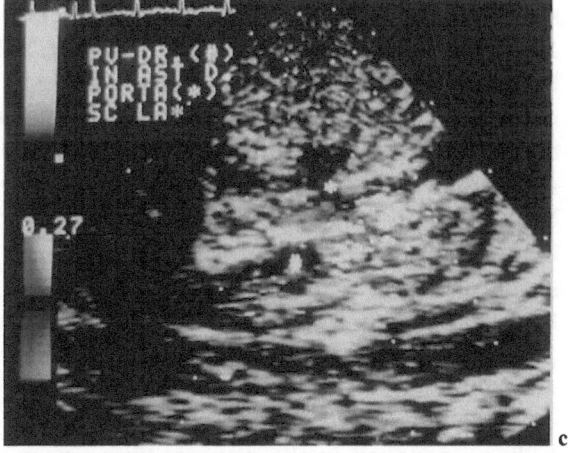

alization is difficult [14, p. 403] but may be much easier with the use of CBFI. We were able to visualize this kind of defect in all four patients whom we have seen so far. Figure 6.8a demonstrates the left-to-right shunt across such a defect together with the anomalous return of the pulmonary veins into the right atrium in the subcostal short axis view.

6.1.5 Anomalous Pulmonary Venous Drainage. Anomalous pulmonary venous connection manifests itself as a pretricuspid left-to-right shunt, therefore its hemodynamics are similar to those of ASDs. There are various forms of anomalous connections of pulmonary veins with the systemic venous system which can be partial or complete.

In Figure 6.8b the drainage of the VCS into the right atrium is shown in a case of partial anomalous pulmonary venous drainage of the supracardiac type. The large flow area in early diastole indicates a strongly increased systemic venous backflow from the upper half of the body, which is especially impressive if compared with the normal flow condition in Fig. 5.11, p. 34. This is suggestive of a supracardiac anomalous pulmonary venous connection and accompanied by right ventricular volume load. The anomalous drainage of pulmonary veins can also be visualized directly using CBFI [61]. Figure 6.8c shows the infradiaphragmatic drainage site in total anomalous pulmonary venous drainage into the portal vein. This connection of the pulmonary veins to the systemic veins was ultimately found after excluding all other possible drainage sites (such as VCS, coronary sinus, or right atrium).

6.1.6 ASD in Combined Heart Disease. ASDs in combined heart disease have already been mentioned (see section 6.1.2) to show the dependency of interatrial shunt patterns on ventricular compliance. Figure 6.9 shows shunts at the *atrial and ventricular levels* occurring at the same time. In Fig. 6.9a, left-to-right shunts across an ASD I, an ASD II (red areas between left and right atria) and simultaneously through a ventricular septal defect (red area in right ventricle) can be seen in late systole. Figure 6.9b shows a left-to-right shunt through an ASD I (red area in left and right atria immediately above the atrioventricular valve level) and at the same time a right-to-left shunt (blue area in right and left ventricles immediately below the atrioventricular valves) across an atrioventricular ventricular septal defect in a case of *endocardial cushion defect,* triggered in late systole. In *complete (D-)transposition of the great arteries* postnatal survival depends on the existence of shunt communications between the pulmonic and systemic circulation where bidirectional exchange of pulmonary and systemic blood can take place. One of the iatrogenic measures which have to be undertaken in the neonate with transposition is the creation or enlargement of an ASD by performing balloon atrioseptostomy [48]. Such an

Fig. 6.9 a, b Simultaneous imaging of atrial and ventricular shunts.
a Left-to-right shunt across three defects: a secundum atrial septal defect *(3)* a primum atrial septal defect *(2)* and a perimembraneous ventricular septal defect *(1)* in late systole in the apical four-chamber view (RBG2). See text for more details

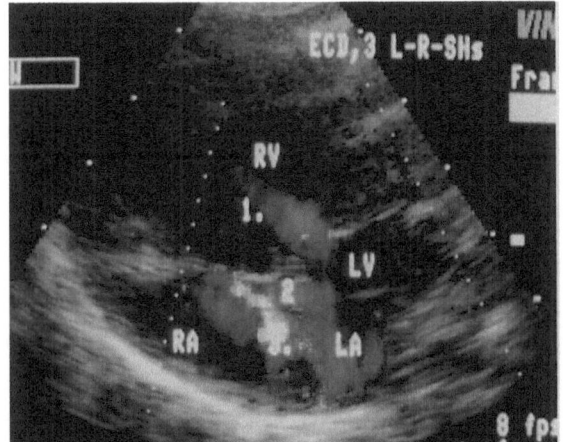

b Left-to-right shunt in late systole across a primum atrial septal defect *(red)* and right-to-left shunt across an inlet ventricular septal defect *(blue)* in a patient with endocardial cushion defect (RB1). See text for more details

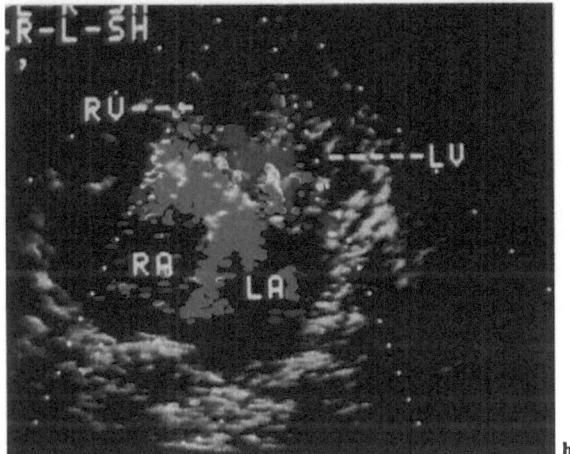

artificially created defect in a neonate, allowing considerable left-to-right shunt in early diastole, is shown in Fig. 6.10a. In Fig. 6.10b the time sequence of the shunt demonstrates that left-to-right shunting (red-yellow) takes the most of the time in the cardiac cycle, as in an uncomplicated ASD (see Fig. 6.4). Pulmonary venous blood is hereby directed into the systemic circulation. At this time, the ductus arteriosus was still patent allowing systemic blood to enter the pulmonic circulation. After the ductus had closed the ASD was the only communication for the exchange of blood between both parts of the circulation. This caused shunting to take place in a bidirectional pattern (Fig. 6.10c) with about equal timing for left-to-right and right-to-left shunting [62]. In *total anomalous pulmonary venous drainage,* pulmonary venous blood returns to the systemic side of the venous system and has to reach the left atrium via an open foramen ovale or an ASD. Figure 6.11 shows the interatrial shunt pattern in a neo-

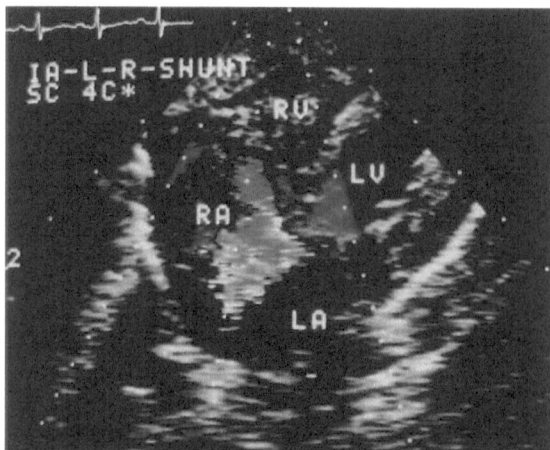

Fig. 6.10a–c Atrial septal defect
in ostium secundum position in
complete transposition of the
great arteries, created by balloon
atrioseptostomy (RBG2).
a Left-to-right shunt across the defect in late systole in the apical
four-chamber view. Left ventricular outflow is colored *blue*

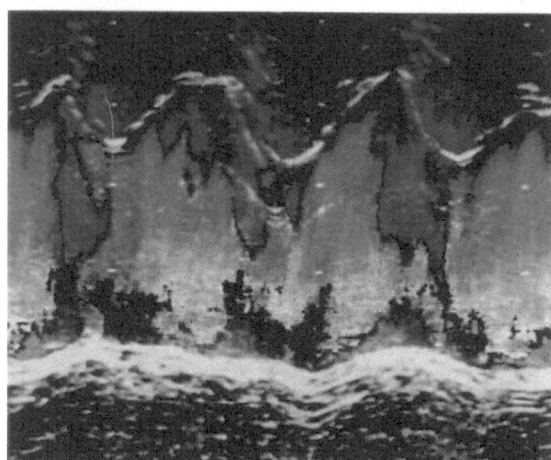

b Time sequence of shunt is demonstrated in the M/Q-mode and
shows left-to-right shunt during
most of the cardiac cycle. See text
for more details

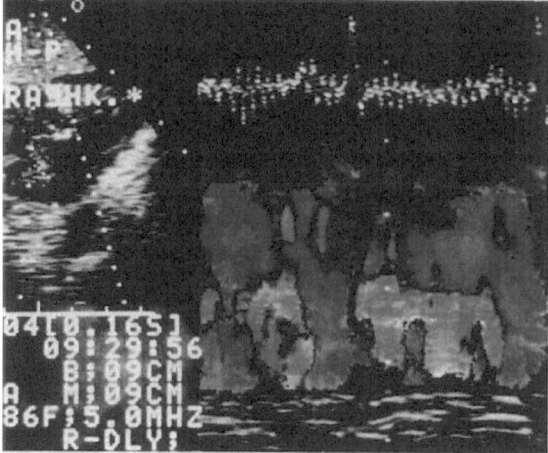

c After spontaneous closure of the
ductus arteriosus, the shunt pattern has changed to bidirectional.
See text for full details

Fig. 6.11 M/Q-mode of shunt in total anomalous pulmonary venous drainage *(TAPVD)* across the atrial septum (RBG2). There is nearly continuous right-to-left shunting which takes place in a turbulent manner because of a restrictive foramen ovale. Insignificant left-to-right shunt *(red)*

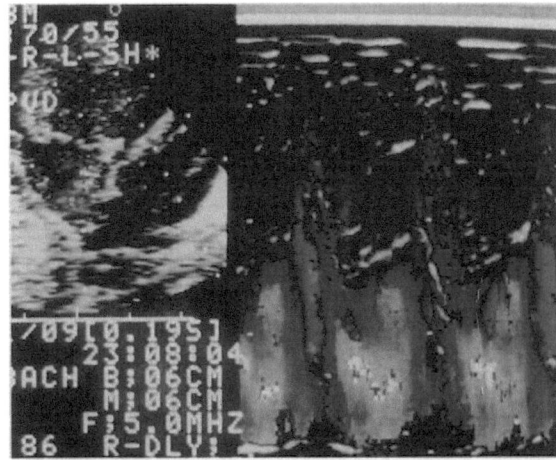

Fig. 6.12 M/Q-mode of vitally important atrial right-to-left shunt in tricuspid atresia (RBG1). There is no flow turbulence indicating that the passage of blood across the atrial septum is unimpeded. Compare with Fig. 6.11

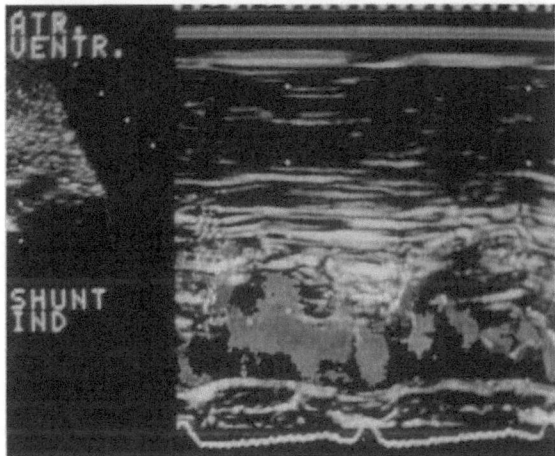

nate with this kind of heart disease: turbulent right-to-left shunting can be seen during most of the cardiac cycle in contrast to which left-to-right shunting is almost negligible.

Atresia of the systemic atrioventricular valve is another example of vitally important right-to-left shunting at the atrial level. An ASD is the only way by which the blood from the caval veins can enter the circulation. In Fig. 6.12 continuous interatrial right-to-left shunt can be seen in a case of tricuspid atresia. A short episode of accidental left-to-right shunt is found in systole.

6.1.7 Diagnostic Pitfalls. Diagnostic pitfalls may occur if the atria are visualized in the subcostal four-chamber view. The backflow from the VCS can easily be mistaken for the left-to-right shunt through an ASD II. This pitfall is avoidable if the atrial septum is visualized additionally in the sub-

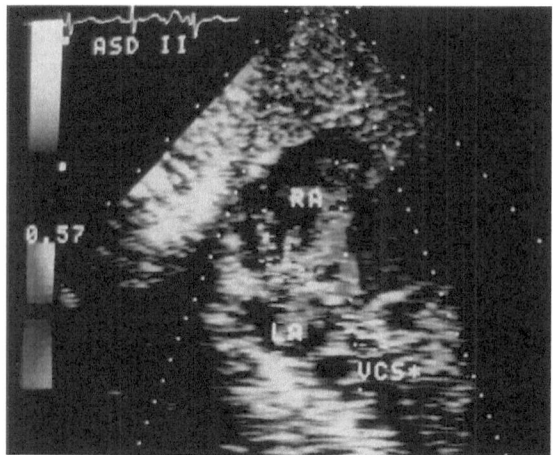

Fig. 6.13 Atrial left-to-right shunt across a secundum atrial septal defect *(ASD II)*, viewed in the subcostal short axis view (RBG2). In this view, the direction of inflowing blood from the superior caval vein *(VCS)* (Fig. 6.8 a) and of atrial shunt *(LA-RA)* are perpendicular to each other. See text for more details

costal short axis view (Fig. 6.13). In this view both flow patterns are easily distinguishable because their flow directions are nearly perpendicular to each other, as can be seen from a comparison of Figures 6.13, and 5.11 (p. 34).

6.2 Shunts at Ventricular Level (Post-tricuspid Shunts – 1 –)

Shunts at ventricular level take place between the high-pressure system of the systemic and the low-pressure system of the pulmonary circulation. Therefore, they occur along a route where there is great difference in systolic pressure, thus leading to a pathological condition with turbulent flow at the wrong location.

6.2.1 Perimembranous Ventricular Septal Defect Including Aneurysm of the Membranous Septum.
Perimembranous ventricular septal defects (VSDs) are the most common VSDs. They are found around the membranous part of the ventricular septum, which consists of a larger interventricular and a smaller atrioventricular part. The latter separates the left ventricle from the right atrium. The left-to-right shunt across perimembranous VSDs is shown at its clearest from the apical position in a view which is between the long axis and the four-chamber views (Fig. 6.14) and may be called "SM view" because it visualizes the septum membranaceum. In Fig. 6.14 three defects with different amounts of left-to-right shunt can be seen, corresponding to the findings during cardiac catheterization. However, in all three cases right ventricular systolic pressure was found to be in the normal range. This implies a relatively high systolic pressure difference between both ventricles causing the shunt to occur as a high-velocity turbu-

Fig. 6.14 a-c Ventricular left-to-right shunt across perimembraneous defects of different sizes. Modified apical four-chamber view (SM view), systolic frame, PRF: 6 kHz (RBG2). Mosaic shunt pattern (see text).
a Small defect (diameter 2 mm), the shunt jet shows only small extension into the right ventricle *(RV)*

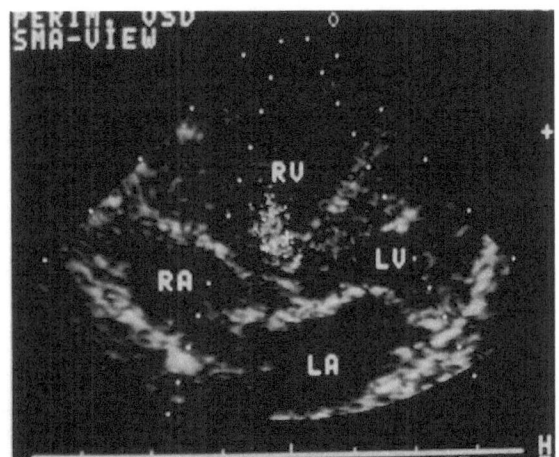

b Medium-sized defect (diameter 3-4 mm) the shunt jet still has a narrow base but reaches the anterior wall of the right ventricle. Convective acceleration in the left ventricle towards the defect can be seen

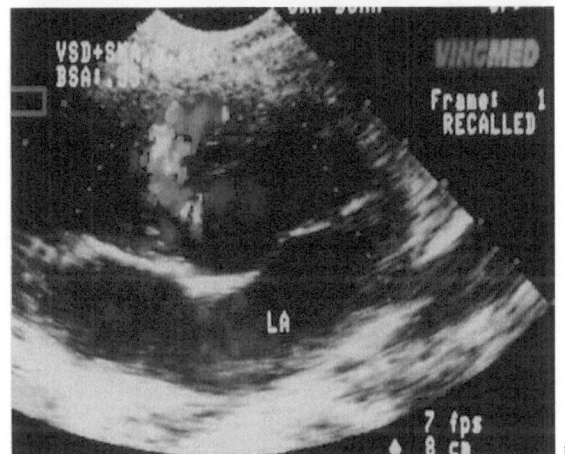

c Moderately large VSD, diameter 4-5 mm. The jet shows a larger base and extends into the right ventricular outflow tract

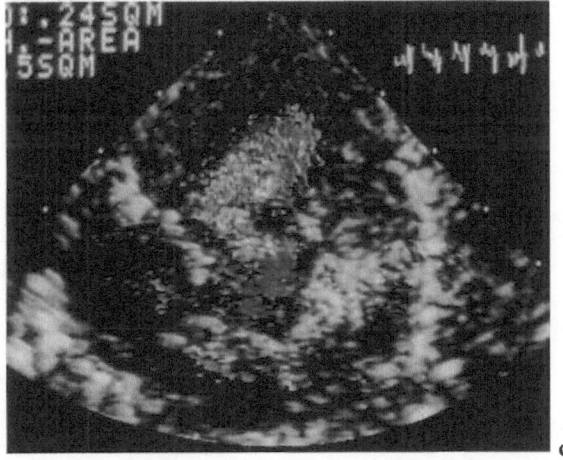

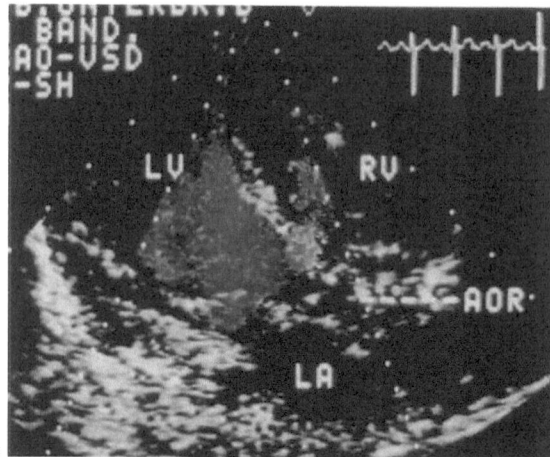

a

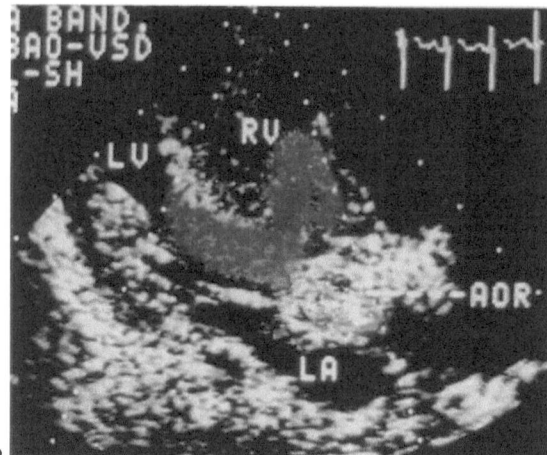

b

Fig. 6.15 a, b Ventricular septal defects *(VSD)* with systolic pressure equalization between the two ventricles after banding of the pulmonary artery. Parasternal long axis view, systolic frame (RBG2). PRF: 6 kHz.
a Left-to-right shunt takes place in a laminar fashion from the left ventricular outflow into the right ventricle. See text for details

b The same defect as in **a** in late diastole shows right-to-left shunt

lent jet. This leads to multiple aliasing and the formation of eddies and vortices imaged as a "mosaic flow pattern."

Figure 6.15 a shows a large defect in the parasternal long axis view which is an appropriate plane for visualization if the defect extends anteriorly below the aortic root. The pattern of left-to-right shunt (Fig. 6.15 a) is completely different from that seen in Fig. 6.14. It is laminar and shows relatively low velocities, indicative of a difference in afterload but not in pressure between the two ventricular cavities, as had been proved by cardiac catheterization in this case. Right-to-left shunt in late diastole is shown in Fig. 6.15 b, the time sequence of bidirectional shunting is demonstrated in Fig. 6.16 b and consists of laminar left-to-right shunt flow in systole and right-to-left shunt flow in diastole. The variations in the time

Fig. 6.16 a-c M/Q-mode of three single ventricular septal defects *(VSD)* with different pressure levels in both ventricles showing the time distribution of the shunt.
a Temporal shunt pattern (RBG2) in a defect with a systolic pressure difference between the two ventricles above 30 mmHg. Left-to-right shunt is starting in late diastole preceded by a short period of right-to-left shunt

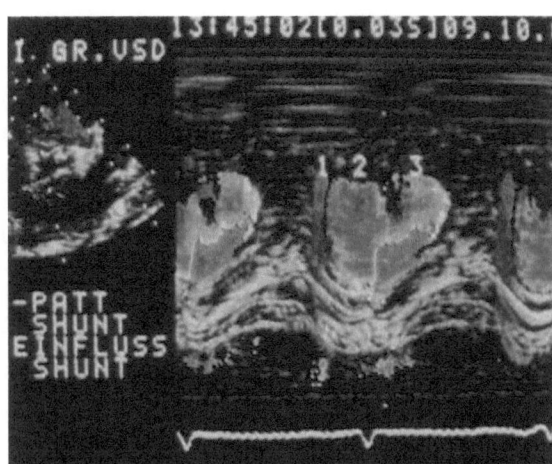

b Shunt in a VSD after banding of the pulmonary artery (RB2). There is systolic pressure equalization between both chambers. The shunt is continuously systolic-diastolic but changes its direction. The *2D insert* shows a period of left-to-right shunt

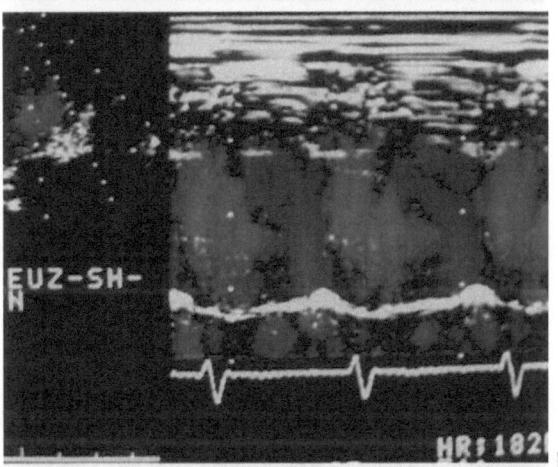

c Shunt in a defect with pulmonary hypertension and increased pulmonary vascular resistance (RBG2). Shunt direction changes 4-6 times during one cardiac cycle: in early systole there is a short period of left-to-right (L-R) shunt interrupted by a short variable phase of right-to-left (R-L) shunt. L-R shunt takes the remaining time of systole. In early diastole there is R-L shunt, atrial contraction leads to L-R shunt which is quickly replaced again by R-L shunt until the cardiac cycle starts again with the next systole. This shunt pattern is different from that described by Kyo [31]

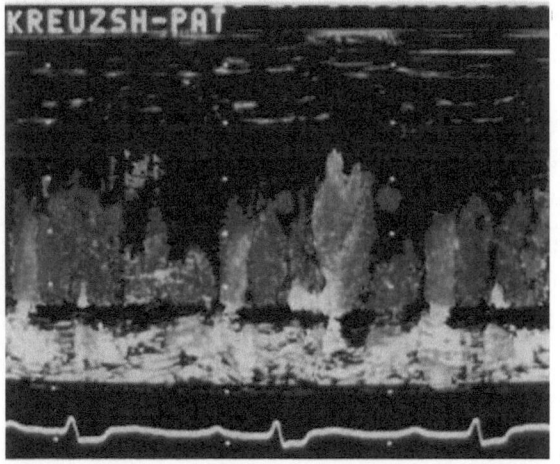

sequence of the shunt patterns in VSDs under different hemodynamic conditions are shown in Fig. 6.16. In defects with considerable pressure difference between the two ventricles (above 30 mmHg), the shunt pattern is almost exclusively left-to-right and may start in late diastole with the onset of atrial contraction after a very short period of right-to-left shunt (Fig. 6.16 a). Shunt velocity increases and causes color aliasing with the beginning of ventricular systole. It stops with the end of systole and starts again as the very short period of right-to-left shunt mentioned above. An increase in shunting volume through a larger defect leads to a change in shunt pattern insofar as the velocity is much lower and the right-to-left shunt (blue in Fig. 6.16 b) takes more time by starting earlier in diastole

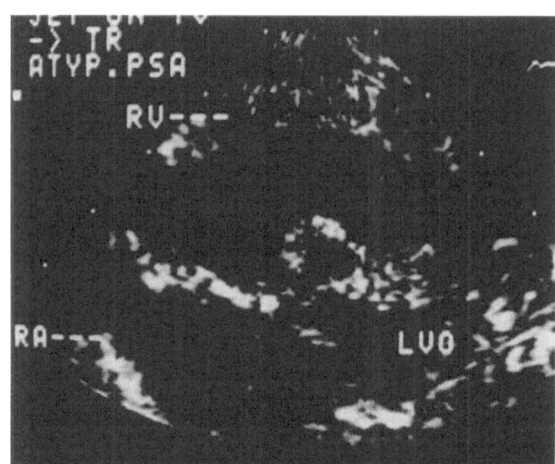

a

Fig. 6.17 a, b Aneurysms of the membranous septum in the apical four-chamber view in systole.
a The aneurysm is bulging from the left ventricular outflow tract *(LVO)* into the right ventricle *(RV)* and is attached to the septal leaflet of the tricuspid valve

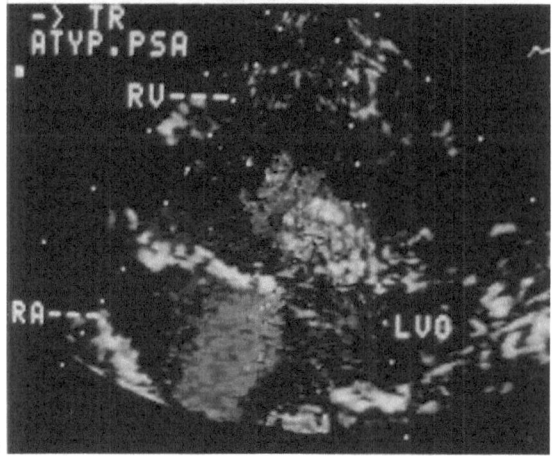

b

b CBFI (RBG2) demonstrates the left-to-right shunt into the right ventricle *(RV)* which occurs in a mosaic pattern indicative of normal systolic RV pressures. Additionally, tricuspid regurgitation *(turquoise)* into the right atrium *(RA)* is visualized representing an infravalvular route of left ventricular-right atrial shunt and also by an extension of left-to-right shunt (red) into early diastole. Shunting occurs as continuously systolic-diastolic throughout the cardiac cycle. If there is a considerable increase in pulmonary vascular resistance, shunting occurs in four to six phases as shown in Fig. 6.16 c [30].

In perimembranous VSDs the formation of *aneurysms* of the membranous septum is a common finding [74]. In systole they bulge into the right ventricle according to the interventricular pressure difference (Fig. 6.17). Their position is immediately distal to the septal leaflet of the tricuspid valve (Fig. 6.17 a) which is sometimes incorporated by forming a tricuspid pouch. This may lead to an incompetence of the tricuspid valve as shown in Fig. 6.17 b and 6.18. The aneurysms may almost completely close the

Fig. 6.18 Aneurysm of the membraneous septum in the apical four-chamber view, systolic frame. The aneurysm has completely occluded the shunt from the left ventricular outflow into the right ventricle *(RV)*. However, a left ventricular-right atrial shunt is clearly indicated by the *turquoise* flow area extending from the attachment of the septal tricuspid valve leaflet into the right atrium *(RA)* (RBG2)

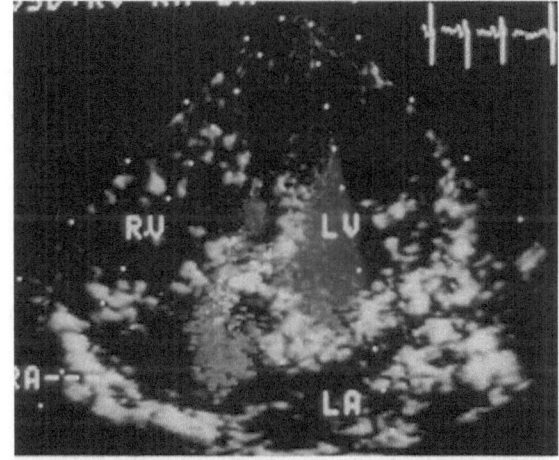

Fig. 6.19 Aneurysm of the membranous septum with residual ventricular septal defect *(VSD)* causing a small amount of left-to-right shunt *(1)* with associated aortic regurgitation *(2)* in the parasternal short axis view (RBG2). Trigger point is the end of isovolumetric relaxation when the septal leaflet of the tricuspid valve *(asterisk)* is just beginning to open as indicated by the *red* hue surrounding its echo structures

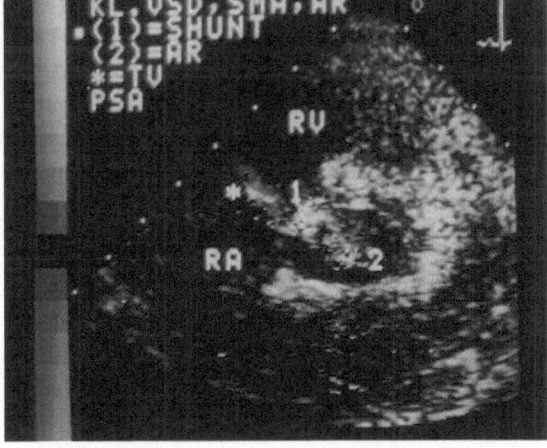

defect, not allowing any significant left-to-right shunting, as shown in Fig. 6.18. Sometimes a membranous defect and/or aneurysm may be complicated by aortic regurgitation caused by a partial or complete prolapse of the right coronary cusp into the left ventricular outflow tract [44]. In Fig. 6.19 a residual VSD with small left-to-right shunt and central aortic regurgitation is imaged.

6.2.2 VSD with Left Ventricular – Right Atrial Shunt. Shunting from the left ventricle into the right atrium may occur directly through a defect of the atrioventricular septum, classified as "a supratricuspid defect" [57], as shown in Fig. 6.18, or via an incompetent tricuspid valve on the infravalvular route, as shown in Fig. 6.20. In our experience, CBFI is more reliable than angiocardiography in detecting a left ventricular-right atrial shunt and in classifying it as supra- or infravalvular. Using continuous wave Doppler the level of communication between the left ventricle and right atrium can be confirmed: direct left ventricular-right atrial communication (supravalvular type) is indicated if the systolic gradient between the left and right ventricles across the VSD is about 20 mmHg below that along the shunt jet from left ventricle into right atrium (Fig. 6.21).

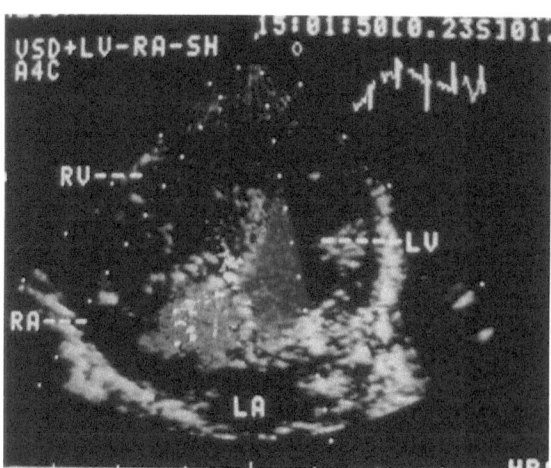

Fig. 6.20 Left-to-right shunt flow across a ventricular septal defect *(VSD)* into the right atrium *(RA)* with direct left ventricular-right atrial communication (supravalvular type) (RBG2). Apical four-chamber view. Comparing this figure with Fig. 6.17b makes it clear that shunts from left to right take place proximal to the insertion of the septal tricuspid leaflet

Fig. 6.21 a Ventricular septal defect with left-to-right shunt into both the right ventricle *(RV, red-yellow)* and the right atrium *(RA, turquoise)*. Apical four-chamber view (RBG2). Two-dimensional imaging does not allow the exact localization of the shunt site as supra- or infravalvular

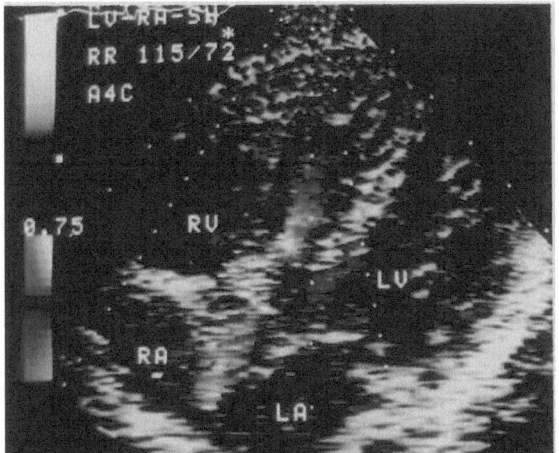

b, c Using continuous wave Doppler measurements the pressure difference along the regurgitant jet into the right atrium (**b**) is calculated to be 68,5 mmHg and that between the two ventrivles (**c**) to be 49 mmHg, which gives a spread of about 20 mmHg between the two values. This proves a direct communication between the left ventricle and the right atrium

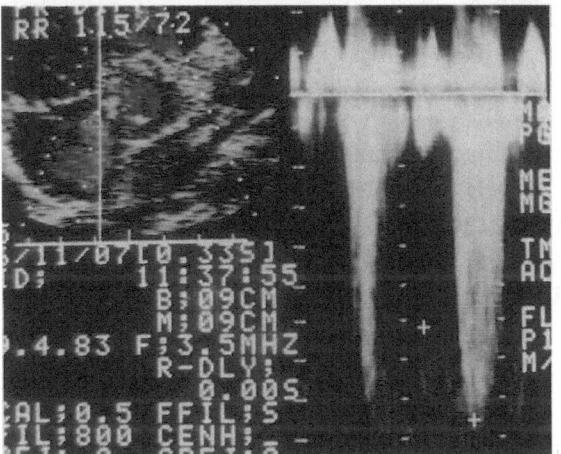

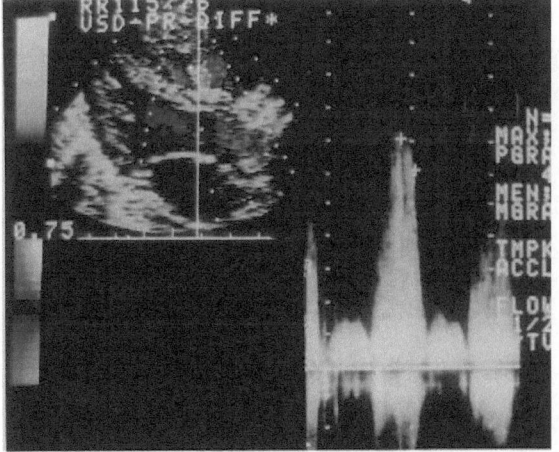

6.2.3 Defects of the Trabeculated Septum. Defects of the trabeculated part of the ventricular septum [65] may occur either in the central part [18] or at the apex. Often they show multiple jets of left-to-right shunting caused either by multiple defects or by crossing of the trabeculae which separate the shunt area into several parts. The central defects are easily recognizable in the short axis views even when they are multiple.

A left-to-right shunt through a small solitary defect is shown in Fig. 6.22 in the subcostal short axis view. This defect was too small to be visualized in the 2D image; the left-to-right shunt, however, can be clearly identified in the cavity of the right ventricle above the anterior papillary muscle.

Two defects in the trabeculated part of the muscular septum are shown in Fig. 6.23. Figure 6.23a shows their position in an apical four-chamber view, the left-to-right shunt is shown in Fig. 6.23b. It is obvious that the diameter of the shunt orifice of the more apically positioned defect is much larger than could be anticipated from the 2D image alone. The reason is that the maximal diameter is not necessarily displayed in the 2D image, whereas this is more probable in the CBFI process because of greater azimuth as a result of greater scan plane thickness (see p. 19).

Defects of the trabeculated septum near the septal-free wall margins [18] cannot be visualized by 2D echo but the left-to-right shunt jet which is directed towards the inflow tract can often be imaged by CBFI as shown in Fig. 6.24.

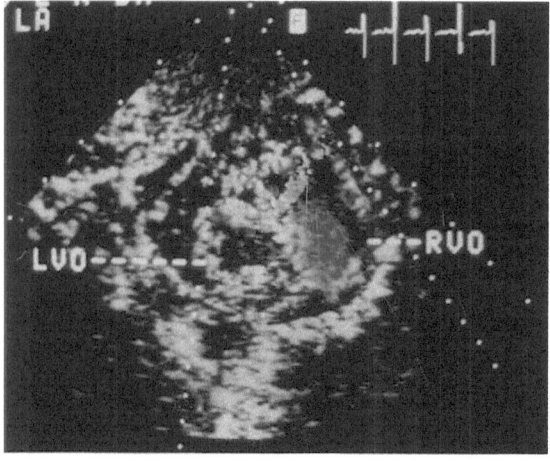

Fig. 6.22 Solitary central defect of the trabeculated ventricular septum in the subcostal short axis view (RBG2). Both ventricles are displayed in the short axis view, the left-to-right shunt is imaged by the *orange-red area* in the right ventricular cavity

Fig. 6.23 a, b Two defects of the trabeculated septum in the apical four-chamber view in systole.
a Two-dimensional display of the ventricular septum in the apical four-chamber view. There are several drop-outs in the septum

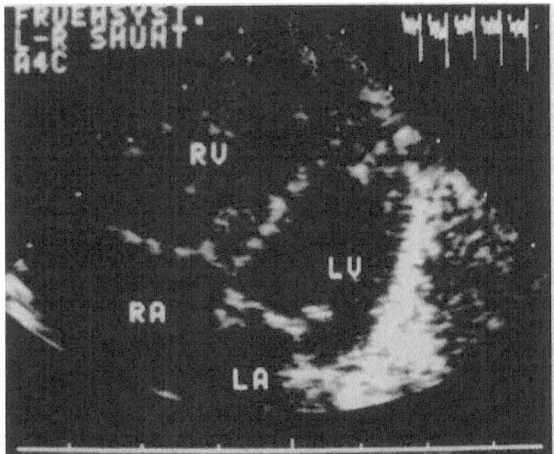

b Two drop-outs are identified with CBFI as defects with left-to-right shunt (RBG2). The discrepancy between the size of the more apically positioned defect in the 2D image and the flow image can be explained by a difference in the azimuth of the sector plane of the two methods. See text for more details

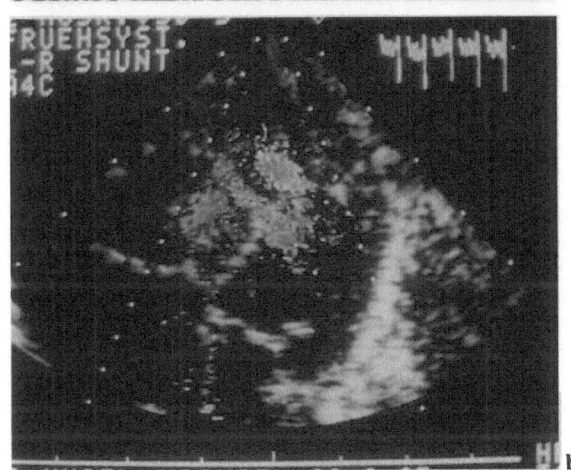

Fig. 6.24 Left-to-right shunt through a marginal defect of the trabeculated ventricular septum is displayed as a flow jet in the right ventricular cavity near the septum with a direction towards the tricuspid valve and therefore displayed in *blue* (RBG2)

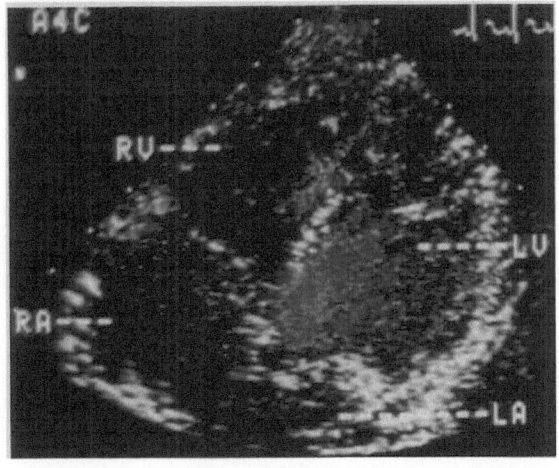

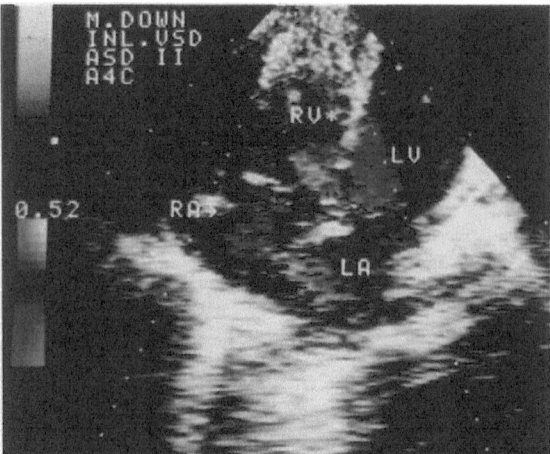

Fig. 6.25 Defect of the inlet part of the ventricular septum in the apical four-chamber view in early systole (RBG2). The left-to-right shunt is displayed in *dark orange*, which is indicative of an elevation of right ventricular pressure near to systemic pressure. There is also a left-to right shunting on atrial level

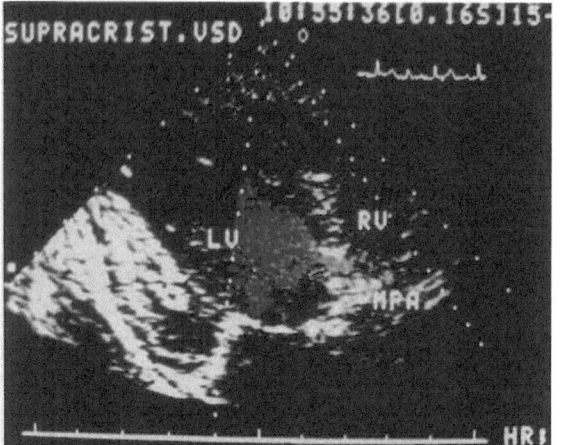

Fig. 6.26a, b Supracristal ventricular septal defect in the parasternal long axis view of the right ventricular outflow tract (**a**) and in the parasternal short axis view (**b**) both in early systole.
a The defect has a diameter of about 4 mm and lies immediately below the pulmonary valve. Left-to-right shunt from the left into the right ventricular outflow tract *(RV)* is turbulent *(cyan)* and is directed towards the posterior leaflet of the pulmonary valve. (RBG2)

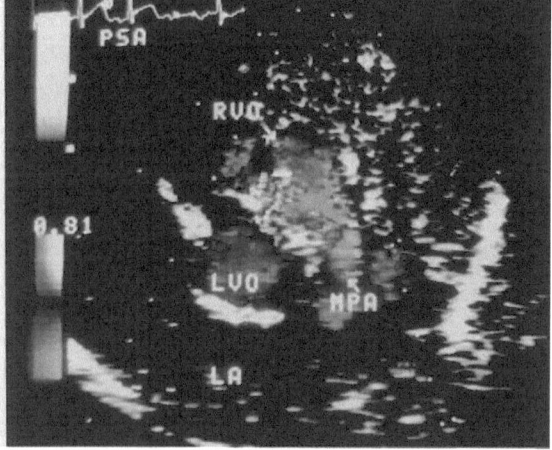

b In the parasternal short axis view the shunt crosses the septum at the right side of the left ventricular outflow tract *(LVO)* at the 2–3 o'clock position (RBG2)

6.2.4 Defects of the Inlet Septum. Defects of the inlet septum are located in the posterior part of the muscular septum near the septal leaflet of the tricuspid valve, slightly anterior to the position of the endocardial cushion defects (see p. 67). The apical four-chamber view is the plane suitable for their visualization, as shown in Fig. 6.25 where a mild tricuspid incompetence can also be seen. The insertion of the atrioventricular valves at the interventricular septum is regular and there is no ASD of the septum primum type, thus excluding an endocardial cushion defect.

6.2.5 Supracristal VSD. Defects of the outlet septum are also termed "supracristal" or "subpulmonary" because of their position immediately below the MPA, as can be seen in Fig. 6.26. In the short axis view their position is distal to the crista supraventricularis on the right side of the left ventricular outflow tract near the 2–3 o'clock position. In our experience this is a very reliable sign for determining their position superior and distal to the crista (Fig. 6.26b).

6.2.6 VSD in Complex Heart Disease. VSDs in combination with other heart diseases have already been shown in Figs. 6.9, p. 51 and 6.25, p. 64. From these figures it is evident that CBFI can show an ASD and a VSD in one image. Figure 6.27 shows right-to-left shunt across a subaortic defect in *truncus arteriosus*. From this figure it is evident that both ventricles empty into the root of the truncus arteriosus. A similar ventricular outflow pattern can be found in cyanotic *tetralogy of Fallot* or in a *double outlet right ventricle*. In these conditions, however, an additional outflow tract leading into the pulmonary artery can be seen in most cases (see Fig. 6.94, p. 112).

Fig. 6.27 Right-to-left shunt across the ventricular septal defect in truncus arteriosus, parasternal long axis view (RBG2). Blood flow from right ventricle *(RV)* and left ventricle *(LV)* is directed into the truncal root *(TA)* which is common to both ventricular cavities. See text for additional details

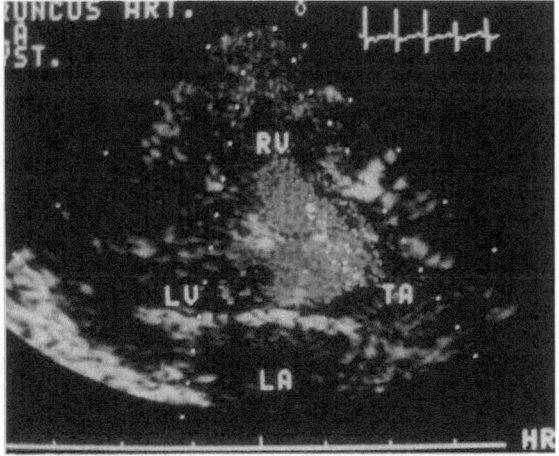

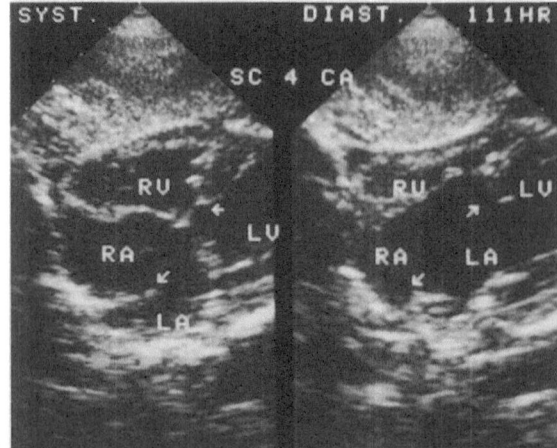

a

Fig. 6.28 a–c Complete atrioventricular canal.
a Morphological aspect in systole *(left)* and diastole *(right)* in the subcostal four-chamber view. A large septum primum atrial septal defect *(between LA and RA)* and a ventricular septal defect *(between LV and RV)* can be seen together with a common atrioventricular valve, which discloses the large common atrioventricular defect in diastole bordered by the rim of the atrial and the ventricular septum *(arrows)*

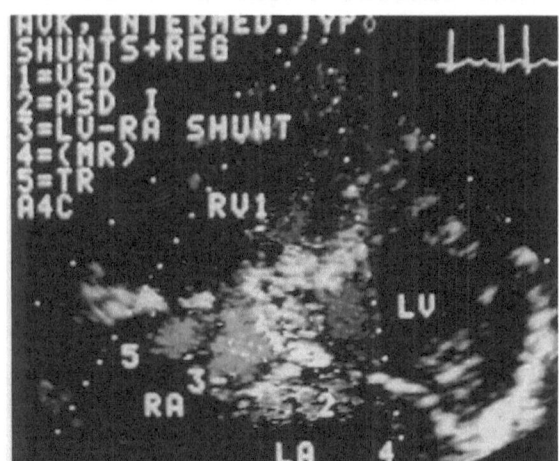

b

b CBFI in systole shows five pathological flow conditions at the same time: 1 left-to-right shunt across the ventricular septal defect; 2 left-to-right shunt across atrial septal defect; 3 left ventricular-right atrial shunt; 4 mitral regurgitation is only partly shown because of limited sector angle; 5 tricuspid regurgitation.

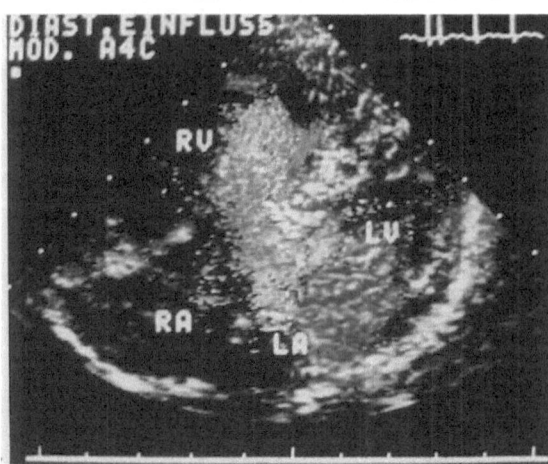

c

c CBFI in early diastole shows that the main inflow is from the left atrium *(LA)* into the right ventricle because of considerable atrial and ventricular left-to-right shunt

In *complete atrioventricular canal* several defects coexist because of incomplete embryological development of the endocardial cushions. The morphological aspect of such heart disease is shown in Fig. 6.28 a. Besides the common atrioventricular valve leaflet, an ASD I and an VSD of the atrioventricular type are visible. Figure 6.28 b shows the systolic flow abnormalities occurring simultaneously. In diastole, the common atrioventricular valve together with the ASD and VSD forms a large, common inflow tract for both ventricular chambers, as can be seen in Fig. 6.28 c.

In *complete (D-)transposition of the great arteries,* the right ventricle is the pumping chamber for the systemic arteries. In the presence of a VSD this will cause an anatomical right-to-left shunt, as is shown in Fig. 6.29. This will take deoxygenated systemical venous blood into the pulmonary artery and help to increase the aortic oxygen saturation.

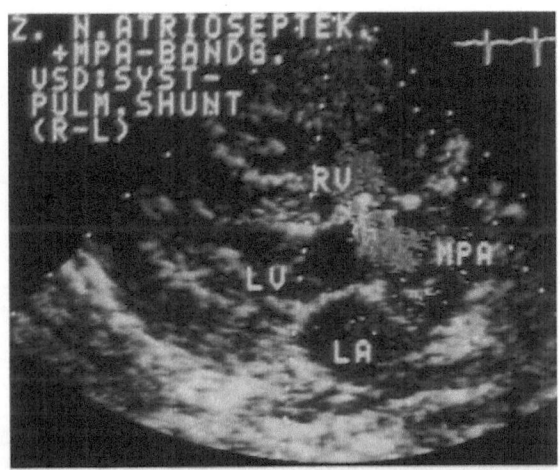

Fig. 6.29 Anatomical right-to-left shunt across a ventricular septal defect *(VSD)* in complete (D-) transposition of the great arteries, parasternal long axis view (RBG2). Blood is flowing away from the right ventricle *(RV)* into the left ventricle *(LV),* which empties into the pulmonary artery *(MPA).* Color aliasing indicates considerably higher pressure in right ventricular cavity

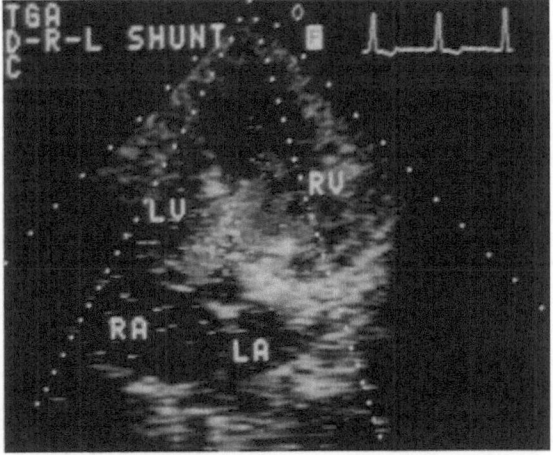

Fig. 6.30 Shunt flow across a ventricular septal defect *(VSD)* in congenitally corrected (L-)transposition in the apical four chamber view from the systemic right ventricle *(RV)* into the pulmonic left ventricle *(LV)* (RBG2). See text for additional details

In *congenitally corrected (L-)transposition* a VSD is common. If there is no pulmonic or subpulmonic obstruction, blood shunts from the systemic (right) ventricle into the pulmonic (left) ventricle, as can be seen in Fig. 6.30. In this situation the hemodynamic effect is the same as in an uncomplicated VSD.

6.2.7 Diagnostic Pitfalls. Pitfalls in the diagnosis of VSDs may occur if the timing and the direction of flow velocities are not observed carefully. Figure 6.31a shows such an example: image T1 shows a left-to-right shunt through a residual VSD after surgical correction of tetralogy of Fallot, the freeze frame was taken 80 ms after R-wave. Image T2 is frozen in diastole (430 ms after R) and shows diastolic inflow into the right ventricle through

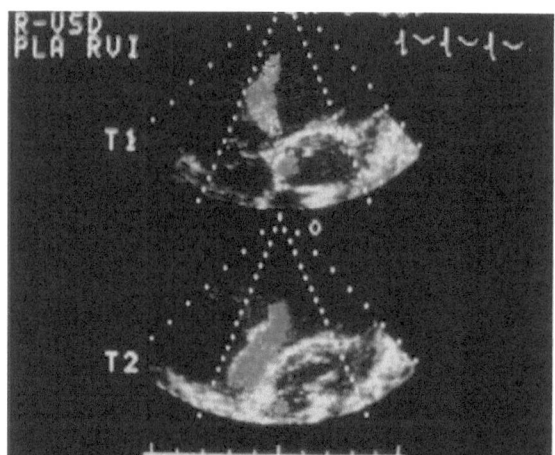

a

6.31a, b Left-to-right shunt across a ventricular septal defect *(T1)* and diastolic inflow through tricuspid valve *(T2)*.
a Ventricular septal defect (VSD) with systolic left-to-right shunt *(T1)* and physiological diastolic inflow into the right ventricle *(T2)*, parasternal short axis view of the left ventricle (RBG2). Both flow events are occurring at the same location. See text for more details

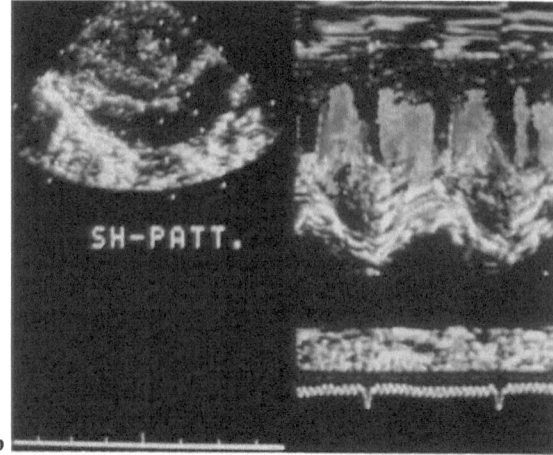

b

b M/Q-mode of the right ventricular inflow (RBG2). Ventricular left-to-right shunt (systolic) and tricuspid valve inflow (diastolic) can be identified with the use of ECG timing

the tricuspid valve, which streams along the septum and is of similar colo-ration as the systolic left-to-right shunt. In Fig. 6.31b an M/Q-mode shows the time course of flow along the interventricular septum during two complete heart cycles. Diastolic inflow across the tricuspid valve and left-to-right shunt across the VSD can be differentiated only by their tim-ing in relation to the ECG. In our experience the existence of a VSD is on-ly proven if it causes systolic turbulence in the right ventricle which can be followed through the septum into the left ventricle, or if in laminar shunt conditions the defect can be visualized by 2D echocardiography alone.

6.3 Shunts at Arterial Level (Post-tricuspid Shunts-2-)

Shunts at arterial level occur between the high-resistance compartment of the systemic circulation and the low-resistance compartment of the pulmo-nary circulation. In small communications this may cause considerable shunt velocities with resulting turbulence and formation of eddies. In larger communications the pressure difference decreases as shunt volume increases even if the pulmonary vascular resistance is still low.

Patent ductus arteriosus (PDA) is by far the most common type of shunt communication on an arterial level. It may persist after birth because there is some deficiency in the normal mechanism of spontaneous closure [17] or it may stay patent because of delayed closure owing to immaturity. The persistence of the ductus arteriosus is found in children born at term whereas a patent ductus arteriosus is common in preterm infants [22]. PDA represents a form of post-tricuspid left-to-right shunt and causes left atrial and left ventricular volume overload. This is reflected by an increase in the ratio of the diameter of the left atrium and the aortic root (LA/AO ratio) which is normally below 1.3 [3, 66]. This parameter is, however, not sufficiently sensitive in our experience nor is it specific for PDA [22].

6.3.1 Persistent or Patent Ductus Arteriosus with Left-to-Right Shunt. Duc-tal left-to-right shunt is best shown in the parasternal short axis view of the great arteries or the long axis view of the PDA from the same position as described earlier [60]. It represents a pathological flow condition which is wrong in time and exhibits turbulent flow. In the case of a *small PDA*, shunting is visible only in diastole and imaged as a small yellow area di-rected from the bifurcation into the proximal MPA while the normal sys-tolic outflow from the right ventricle is displayed in blue. In most cases the shunting jet runs along the superior wall of the MPA (Fig. 6.32a). Some-times, however it is directed towards the posterior wall and crosses the lu-men of the pulmonary artery (Fig. 6.32c). It may also reach the pulmonary

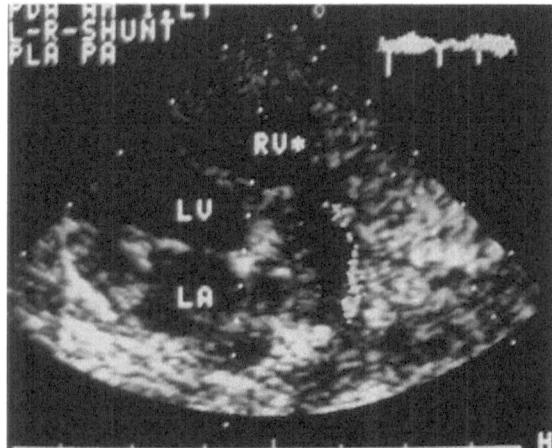

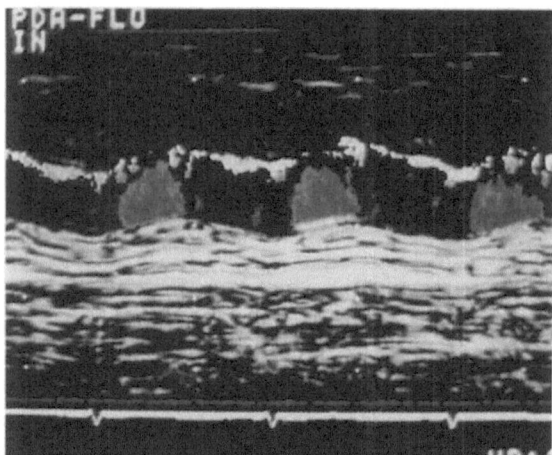

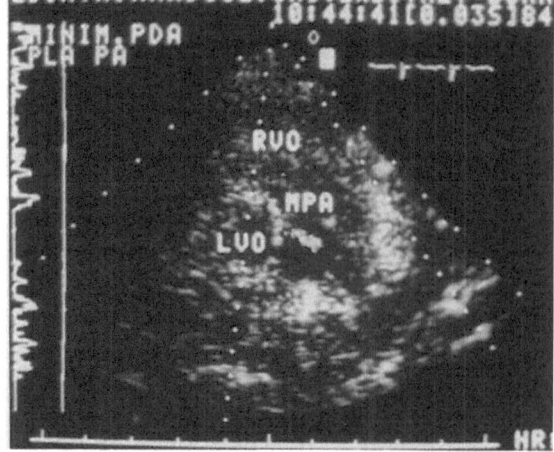

Fig. 6.32 a–c Small amount of ductal left-to-right shunt, (RBG2). **a** Small left-to-right shunt is visualized in the parasternal long axis view of the pulmonary artery as a *yellow* jet in diastole at the superior wall of the main pulmonary artery and it extends down to the pulmonic valve where it can be picked up by the M/Q-mode (see **b**)

b M/Q-mode of small ductal left-to-right shunt of **a** at the level of the pulmonic valve, picked up at the anterior part of the pulmonic valve. The shunt jet is very small thus forming only a thin *yellow line* which is interrupted in systole by the outflow into the pulmonary artery *(blue)* from the right ventricle

c Atypical jet direction of a small ductus arteriosus towards the posterior wall of the pulmonary artery in the parasternal long axis view

valve where it can be picked up by the M/Q-mode (Fig. 6.32 b). In systole the jet is pushed towards the wall of the MPA by the blood ejected on the normal route from the right ventricle (Fig. 6.32 b). This happens despite the fact that the pressure difference between the descending aorta and the MPA is highest in early systole and may be due to the relatively small shunt volume of the ductus in comparison to the large right ventricular outflow volume.

A *medium-sized ductus* is characterized by a larger shunt area in the MPA, as shown in Fig. 6.33 a. Nevertheless, it is still difficult to visualize the left-to-right shunt in systole when the right ventricular blood enters the pulmonary artery. In the M/Q-mode the jet can be followed deeper into the MPA because of its larger diameter (Fig. 6.33 b).

A *large ductal left-to-right shunt* is easily visualized in systole together with the normal orthograde outflow, in diastole it fills the MPA complete-

Fig. 6.33 a, b Medium-sized ductal left-to-right shunt into MPA (RBG2).
a Diastolic frame, the jet occupies more space within the MPA than in Fig. 6.32 a, c. The planimetered area is a semiquantitative measure for the size of the shunt in premature babies, (RBG2). See text for more information

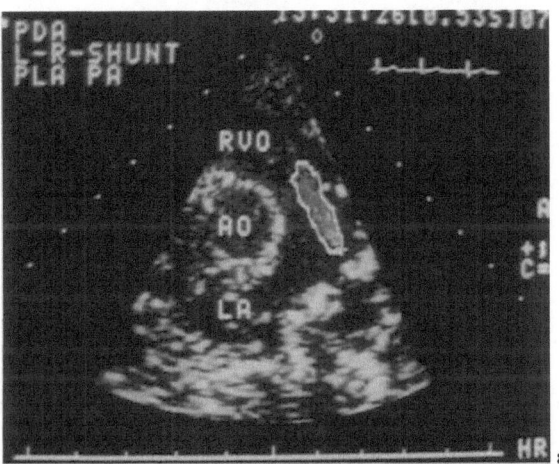

b Shunt pattern of a medium-sized ductus. The jet line in the M/Q-mode is larger than in Fig. 6.32 b

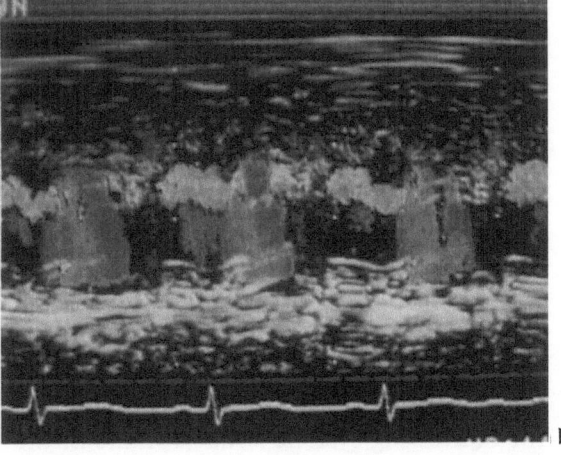

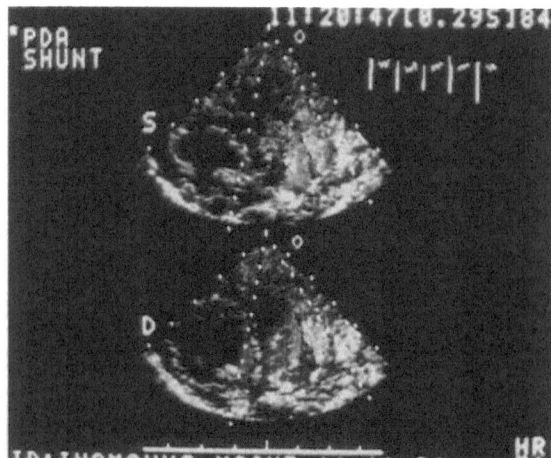

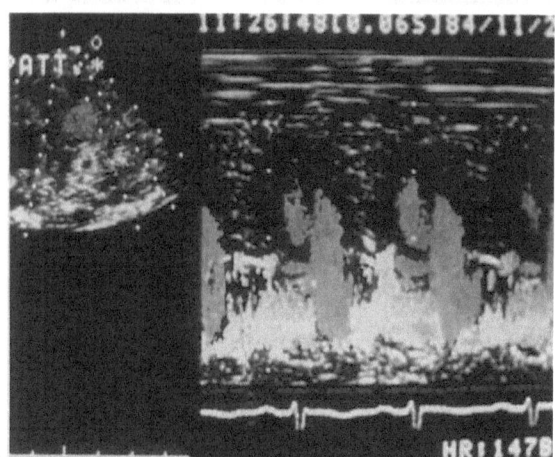

Fig.6.34a, b Large left-to-right shunt across a ductus (RBG2).
a In systole *(upper frame, S)* ductal left-to-right shunt *(yellow)* represents enough volume of blood to hold against the normal outflow into MPA *(blue)*. In diastole *(lower frame, D)* the shunting blood flow *(yellow)* fills nearly the whole MPA. Both frames were taken in the parasternal long axis view of the MPA

b M/Q-mode performed through the inferior parts of MPA shows that the whole depth of the MPA is filled almost completely by shunting blood flow from the bifurcation to the pulmonic valve *(yellow)* in diastole. In this inferior part of the MPA systolic outflow *(blue)* is pushing ductal shunting flow almost down to the bifurcation

ly from the bifurcation to the valve (Fig.6.34a, upper frame). Additionally a blue field can be seen (diastolic frame in Fig.6.34a) and this represents shunted blood rebounding from the pulmonary valve. This flow pattern is indicative of a large systolic-diastolic shunt volume in the presence of a considerable systolic-diastolic pressure difference across the PDA. In the M/Q-mode the jet fills nearly the entire depth of the MPA (Fig.6.34b).

In *uncomplicated* ductuses the left-to-right shunt is continuously systolic-diastolic. If the shunt volume is small-to-moderate, the jet has to give way to the normal systolic outflow from the right ventricle (blue in Figs.6.32b, 6.33b, 6.34b) and is deflected into the marginal parts of the pulmonary artery which are usually near the superior wall. In the case of a large ductus, the shunt volume represents enough mass to hold out against the outflowing systolic stroke volume of the right ventricle (Fig.6.34a).

In our experience the *diagnostic accuracy* of CBFI is excellent. In a study group of 72 infants and children a ductus was diagnosed in 30 patients and confirmed by catheterization or operation, in two patients the typical ductal left-to-right shunt could not be visualized. Both had large shunts at the atrial and ventricular levels resulting in pulmonary hypertension. This resulted in the absence of a significant pressure difference across the ductus and thus prevented the typical shunt jet from building up. Diagnostic sensitivity was 96%. There was no false-positive diagnosis of PDA, giving a specificity of 100%. In order to get a *quantitative idea* about the ductal shunt, we measured the maximal visible area occupied by the diastolic left-to-right shunt by planimetry, as shown in Fig. 6.33 a [33]. This was performed in 33 premature babies born between week 25 and 35 (mean: 31), weighing 1020–2500 g (mean: 1520 g). The measured area was expressed in square centimeters and normalized by division of the body weight (in kilograms). The correlation with the LA/AO ratio derived from the M-mode as the only quantitative hemodynamic parameter available in all patients is shown in Fig. 6.35. The results of the linear correlation are

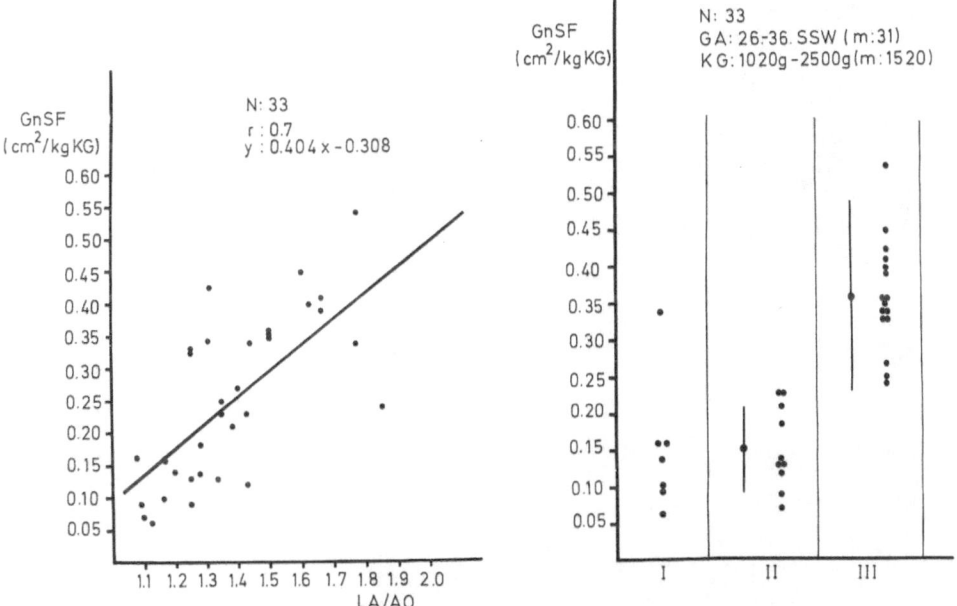

Fig. 6.35 Correlation between area of ductal left-to-right shunt in pulmonary artery, normalized for body weight *(GnSF)* and LA/AO ratio. See text for more details

Fig. 6.36 Relationship of left-to-right shunt velocity area in pulmonary artery in diastole. normalized for body weight *(GnSF)* and clinical outcome of 33 premature infants. Except for one case all the premature infants who had to undergo ductal closure had an area above 0.24 cm²/kg body weight. The one exception was a premature infant in the 2nd day of life. *I*, No signs of cardiac failure; *II*, cardiac failure manageable by conservative treatment; *III*, cardiac failure could only be managed by ligation of the ductus arteriosus

unsatisfactory. However, when we compared the normalized ductal shunt area with the clinical outcome, it became evident that all but one of the premature babies in whom the area was above 0.24 cm²/kg had to undergo closure of the ductus for clinical reasons [33] (Fig. 6.36). From this we conclude that the shunt area may give a new prognostic parameter for early indication of ductal closure beyond the 2nd day of life before the dramatic and dangerous clinical picture of heart failure develops. Prospective studies on this parameter are currently being undertaken by our group.

6.3.2 PDA with Right-to-Left Shunt. Ductal right-to-left shunt is found in conditions with *high pulmonary vascular resistance* if there is persistent patency of the ductus arteriosus. This flow condition is, however, difficult to image because flow velocities in the pulmonary artery do not exhibit any major changes from normal and because in most cases there is no detect-

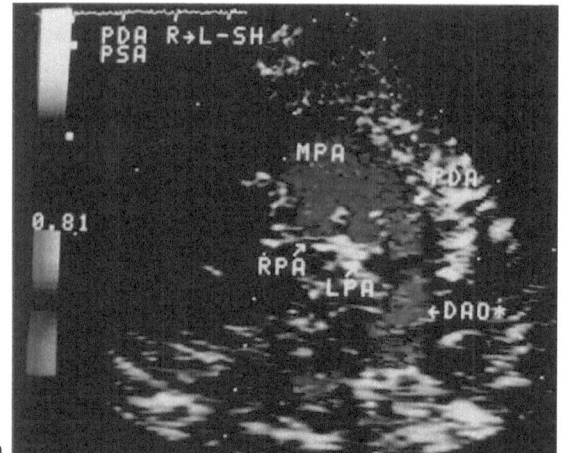

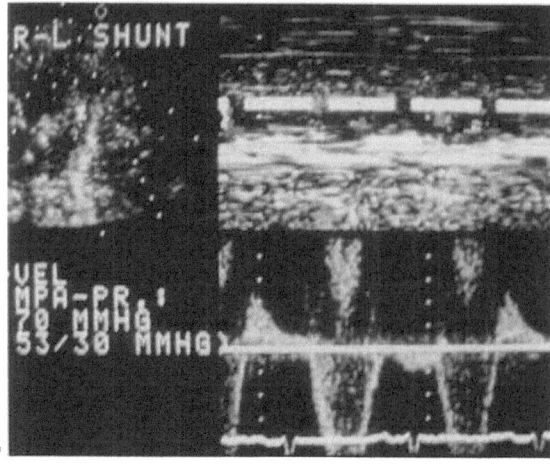

Fig.6.37a, b Mid-systolic right-to-left shunt across a patent ductus arteriosus in a neonate with persistent fetal circulation.
a Normal systolic outflow *(blue)* continues across the patent ductus arteriosus into the descending aorta *(DAO)* in the parasternal long axis view of the pulmonary artery (RBG2)

b Shunt across PDA, sample volume is positioned in the ductus. It starts in mid-systole and extends into diastole until the P-wave appears

able turbulence. Therefore, the ductus and its connection to the descending aorta have to be visualized directly and their flow pattern has to be picked up, as shown in Fig. 6.37a. Using the M/Q-mode and single gate Doppler, as shown in Fig. 6.37b, the accurate timing of the shunt can be judged. It starts fairly late in systole and extends into diastole. Additionally, systolic pressure in the pulmonary artery can be determined noninvasively by measuring the systolic and diastolic ductal flow velocities, calculating from these the pressure differences according to the simplified Bernoulli equation [23], and adding these values to the systolic or diastolic blood pressure values obtained by the Riva-Rocci method at the right arm.

6.3.3 PDA in Complex Heart Disease.
In complex heart disease the ductus arteriosus plays an ambiguous role: in the case of increased pulmonary perfusion it may contribute considerably to the amount of left-to-right

Fig. 6.38 a, b Ductus-dependent heart disease shown in infantile preductal coarctation.
a Systolic right-to-left shunt across a PDA, which has been reopened by prostaglandin, from the MPA into the descending aorta *(DAO)* in iuxtaductal coarctation. Parasternal short axis view (RBG2)

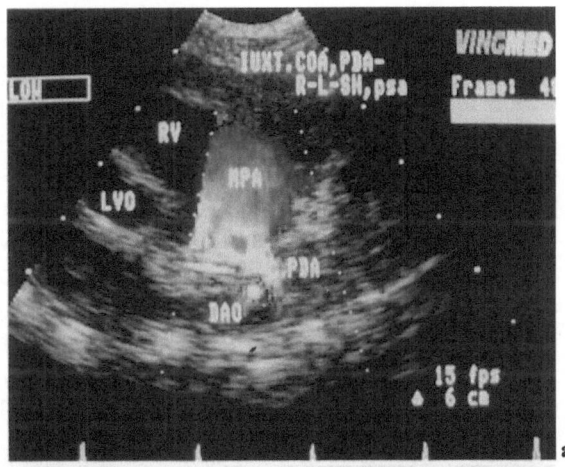

b Systolic MPA flow velocities in a neonate with critical pulmonic stenosis, parasternal short axis view (RBG2). The MPA shows predominantly retrograde flow *(red)* because the ductus arteriosus has been reopened by prostanglandin and is perfusing most of the MPA

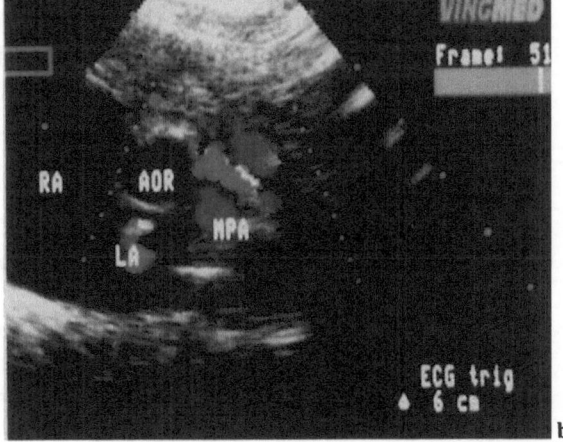

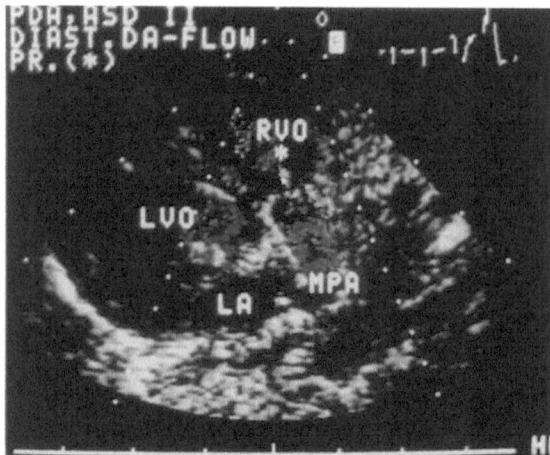

Fig. 6.39 Diastolic frame of main pulmonary artery *(MPA)* in late diastole, parasternal position (RBG2). Left-to-right shunt into the main pulmonic artery across a ductus is shown *(yellow)* as well as pulmonic valve regurgitation into the right ventricular outflow tract *(RVO asterisk)*. The *blue* flow in MPA is away-flow of shunted blood into the peripheral pulmonary arteries

shunt, in cases with diminished lung perfusion it may be the only source of blood supply to the pulmonary arterial system. Together with defects which lead to a critically decreased perfusion of the systemic circulation *(hypoplastic left heart syndrome, preductal coarctation)* they form the group of the so-called ductus-dependent heart diseases. In many of these infants, patency of the ductus must be restored by infusion of prostaglandin E_1 or E_2 to maintain the circulation. Fig. 6.38a was taken in a neonate with iuxtaductal coarctation under the infusion of prostaglandins which re-opened the PDA thus allowing right-to-left shunt from the MPA into the descending aorta. In *high-degree pulmonic stenosis* or *atresia*, the pulmonary arterial flow is dependent upon the left-to-right shunt across the ductus arteriosus. Such a case is shown in Fig. 6.38b.

6.3.4 Diagnostic Pitfalls. Pitfalls in the diagnosis of a left-to-right shunt across a PDA may occur if the flow pattern is not carefully observed. In Fig. 6.101 (p. 116) diastolic backflow in the MPA, caused by incompetence of the pulmonic valve, can be observed. The finding of pulmonic regurgitation itself, however, does not exclude a PDA, since both lesions often co-exist (Fig. 6.39).

6.4 Abnormalities of the Left Ventricular Inflow

Different kinds of congenital and acquired heart diseases, which cause an alteration in the blood flow pattern in the left ventricular inflow tract, are included in this section. Stenoses lead to flow abnormalities which are characterized by the appearance of pathologically high velocities at regular diastolic timing. Regurgitations cause systolic flow disturbances to appear at the wrong moment and show high velocities with alias and disturbed systolic flow. Both types of pathological flow pattern can be seen in combined mitral valve disease and may be recorded in one trace by using the M/Q-mode.

6.4.1 Mitral Stenosis. Mitral stenosis is characterized by a typical diastolic flow pattern in the 2D display which is reminiscent of a candle flame (Figs. 6.40–6.42). The jet velocities reach a maximum of about 2 m/s [19, p. 111] in the left ventricle, which is a relatively low value compared to stenotic lesions of the arterial valves. Therefore the amount of turbulence within the jet is relatively small even in a high-degree stenosis. With increasing severity, the diameter of the jet decreases and the area of aliasing within the jet occupies relatively more space, as can be seen in Fig. 6.42.

Measurement of the mitral valve orifice may be more correct if the cross-sectional area of the jet rather than the valve opening area is determined. The reason for this is that it may be difficult to visualize the real orifice because of technical difficulties (appropriate gain settings, problems of lateral resolution, adjustment of the transducer to the right plane, etc.) or because very strong echoes arising from calcification of the leaflets artificially reduce the measurable orifice in the conventional 2D image [36, 37]. The jet diameter remains practically the same over a considerable dis-

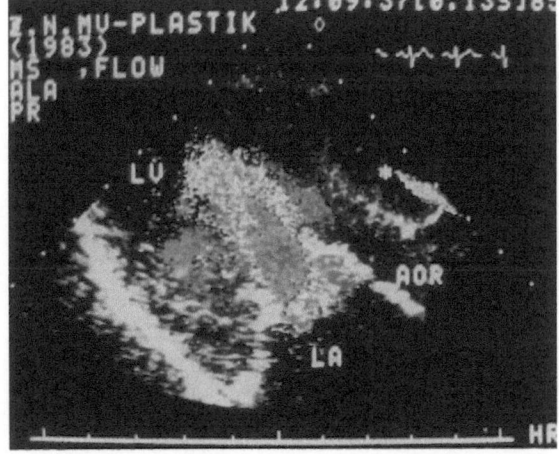

Fig. 6.40 Mild mitral stenosis after surgical reconstruction of a congenital mitral cleft, apical long axis view (RBG2) PRF: 6 kHz. Inflow area in early diastole has a relatively large diameter, *blue* area of color aliasing is confined to the left ventricular inflow and does not reach far into the left ventricular cavity. Streamline separation is indicated by the backflow *(blue)* behind the posterior leaflet. The asterisk (*) is marking slight pulmonic regurgitation

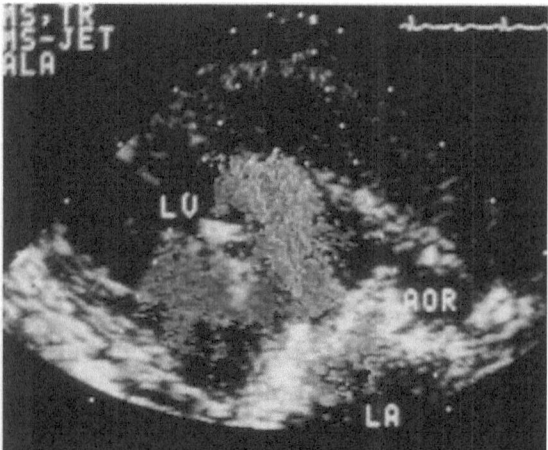

Fig. 6.41 Moderately severe mitral stenosis caused by a stenotic homograft in mitral position, apical long axis view (RBG2), PRF: 6 kHz. The diameter of the late diastolic flow area is considerably smaller than in Fig. 6.4, the *blue* area of aliasing representing the core of the jet reaches down to the apical part of the interventricular septum

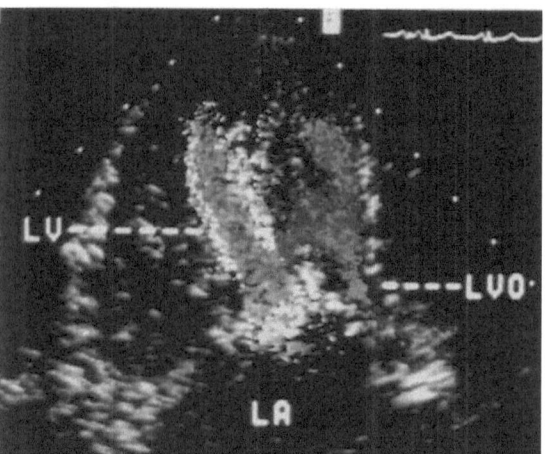

Fig. 6.42 Severe mitral stenosis caused by rheumatic heart disease (combined with mitral regurgitation). Late diastolic inflow, apical long axis view (RBG2) PRF: 6 kHz. The inflow area has a relatively small diameter and is largely occupied by an aliased *blue* color indicating that most of the inflow exceeds the Nyquist level of 3 MHz which is equal in this projection to 69 cm/s

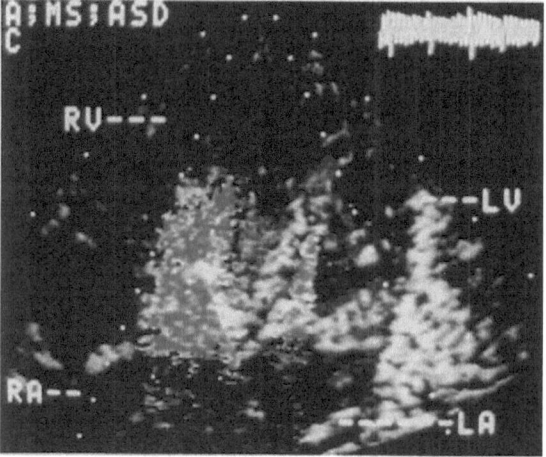

Fig. 6.43 Congenital mitral stenosis in an infant, apical four-chamber view (RBG2) PRF: 6 kHz. Despite considerable narrowing of the mitral valve opening area the typical "candle flame" is missing. See text for more details

tance from the mitral orifice into the left ventricle (Figs. 6.41, 6.42) so that measurement of the orifice may be performed distal to the free edges of the mitral valve with fewer technical difficulties and without disturbances from structural interferences.

Congenital mitral stenosis in infancy may present itself in a different way, as can be seen in Fig. 6.43. The typical "candle flame" within the left ventricle is missing, and from this it is obvious that the diastolic flow velocities across the mitral valve are in the physiological range. The reason is that the left atrium is decompressed by the incompetence of the foramen ovale, and this leads to a left-to-right shunt across the atrial septum and lowers the diastolic transmitral pressure gradient to normal values. However, the hemodynamic situation is reflected by a considerable difference in the diameters of both atrioventricular flow areas indicating a much higher volume flow rate through the tricuspid than through the mitral valve.

Diagnostic pitfalls are not liable to occur in mitral stenosis. In severe mitral regurgitation a relative stenosis may cause a candle flame imaging of diastolic inflow. However, the base of the jet at the mitral orifice is relatively large as compared to organic stenosis (Fig. 6.40).

6.4.2 Mitral Regurgitation. The diagnosis of mitral incompetence is one of the domaines of CBFI. In the short time since CBFI has become available it has proved to be especially valuable for qualitative and semiquantitative diagnosis of regurgitations [24, 43]. The regurgitant flow is characterized by high velocities and turbulence occurring at the wrong time during the cardiac cycle (Fig. 6.44). In mild-to-moderate incompetence the regurgitant jet shows a narrow base originating at the site of leakage which is situated between the commissures of both mitral leaflets (Figs. 6.45 a, b). In more severe insufficiencies, systolic regurgitant flow fills nearly the whole cavity of the left atrium thereby hiding the site of the leak (Fig. 6.45 c). In such a case, the leakage may be visualized from the ventricular side of the mitral valve, as can be seen in Fig. 6.46 which shows the typical "reversed Y-sign" in systole [41, p. 55]. Sometimes two regurgitant jets can be observed, as shown in Fig. 6.47.

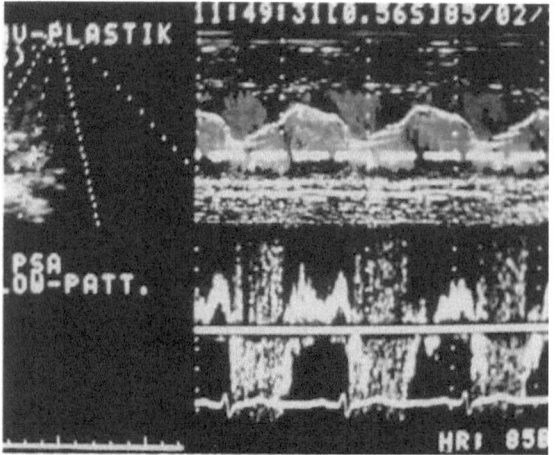

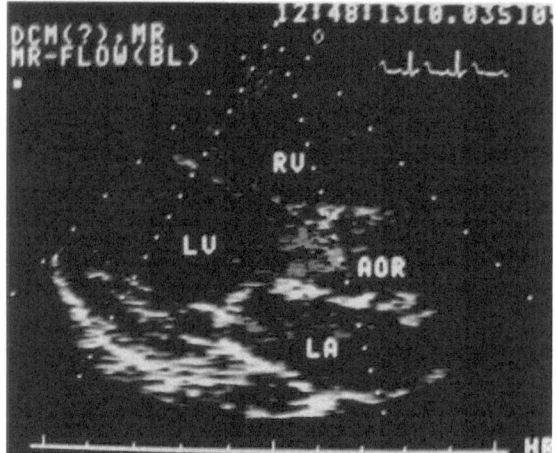

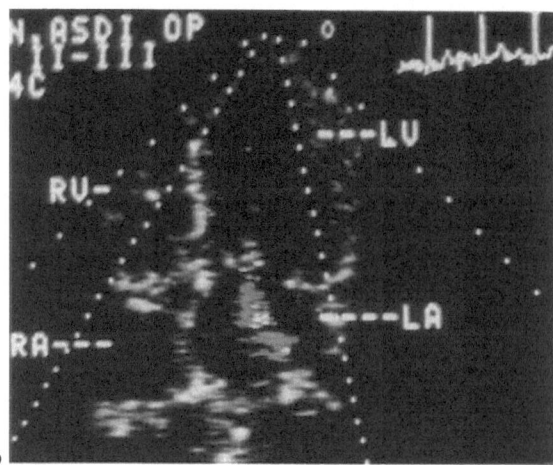

Fig. 6.44 Mitral regurgitation displayed by all three modalities of pulsed Doppler. CBFI *(upper left)* shows the 2D distribution of regurgitation flow in the left atrium. The *dotted line* in the color sector indicates the location from which the M/Q-mode *(upper right)* is derived. The latter shows the temporal distribution of normal *(red-orange)* and pathological *(turquoise)* transmitral flow as well as the normal left ventricular outflow *(blue)* over the whole depth of investigation. The *interrupted horizontal line* within the M/Q-mode defines the location of the sample volume from which the FFT trace *(lower right)* is recorded. From the trace it is obvious that the systolic regurgitant flow is turbulent, as indicated by the *turquoise* color in both the M/Q-mode and CBFI image as well as by spectral broadening in the FFT trace

Fig. 6.45 a–c Slight-to-moderate mitral regurgitations (RBG2).
a Slight mitral incompetence in the parasternal long axis view, the area of turbulent regurgitant flow in the left atrium *(LA)* is only small and does not reach far back into the cavity in this case of dilative cardiomyopathy

b Moderately severe mitral incompetence after sirgucal closure of an atrial septal defect *(ASD)* in the apical four-chamber view. The regurgitant jet extends to the posterior atrial wall but does not occupy a large area of the LA section

c Severe mitral regurgitation causing the regurgitant backflow to fill
most of the left atrium in the apical long axis view

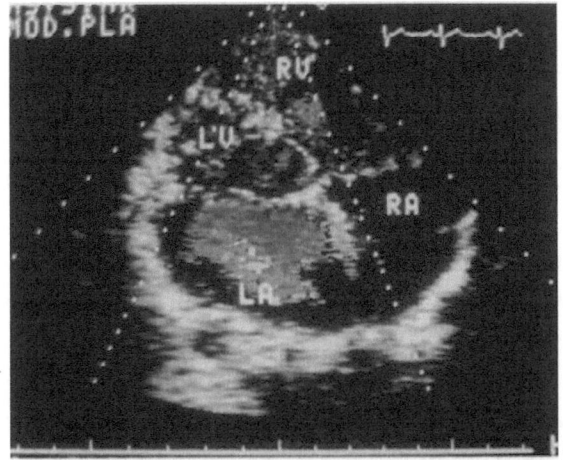

Fig. 6.46 Severe mitral incompetence in the apical long axis view
(RBG2). Outflow from the left
ventricle *(LV)* takes place at two
sites thereby creating the "reversed Y-sign:" one route leads
into the aortic route *(AOR)*, the
other one across the severely incompetent mitral valve into the
left atrium *(LA)* where the regurgitant flow is not displayed in this
particular sectional plane. There
are some flow velocities *(red-
orange)* from the pulmonary veins

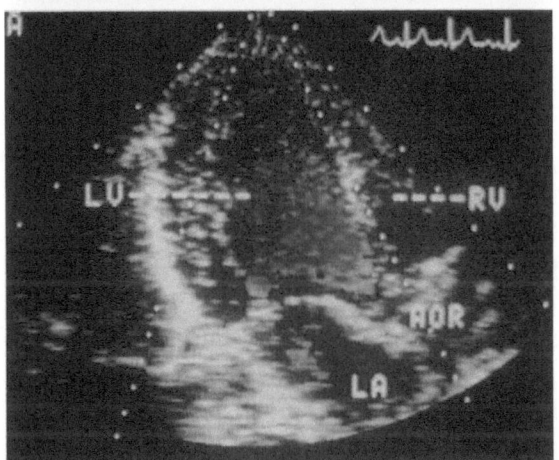

Fig. 6.47 Mitral regurgitation giving rise to two jets in the left atrium *(LA)* after surgical correction
of complete atrioventricular canal,
apical four-chamber view (RBG2)
The *red meandering line* indicates
the build-up time of a CBFi-
frame. The *last complete square* on
the right side shows duration and
timing of the picture

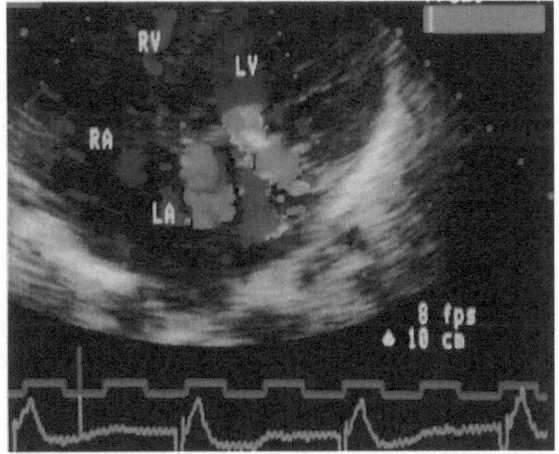

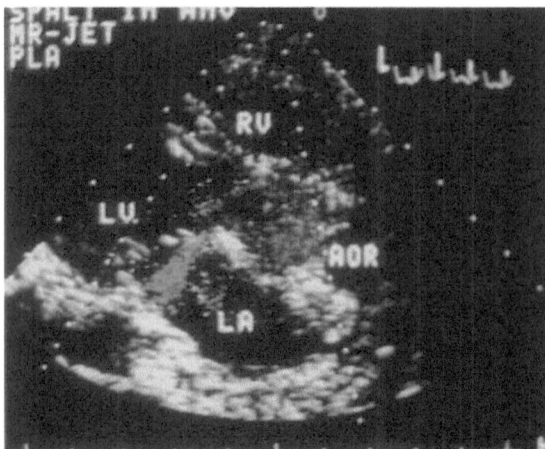

Fig. 6.48 Congenital mitral incompetence caused by a cleft in the anterior mitral leaflet, parasternal long axis view (RBG2). The regurgitant jet *(turquoise)* is entering the left atrium *(LA)* in an oblique fashion from the middle part of the anterior mitral leaflet and splashing against the posterior wall near the posterior leaflet

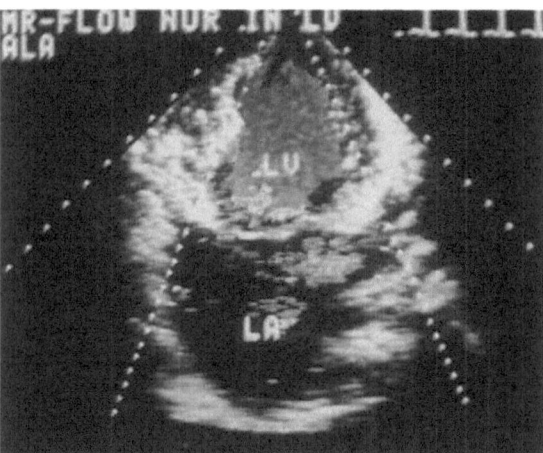

Fig. 6.49 Very severe mitral incompetence with giant left atrium (RBG2). Convective acceleration of left ventricular *(LV)* blood towards the mitral valve with aliasing to *orange-yellow* can be seen in the apical long axis view. In the giant left atrium *(LA)*, however, the regurgitant jet is not visible and there are only some eddies

Congenital mitral regurgitation may be caused by a cleft in the anterior mitral valve leaflet [10]. In such a case the regurgitant jet originates from the anterior mitral leaflet and splashes in an oblique direction into the left atrium (Fig. 6.48).

The *quantification* of mitral regurgitation by CBFI has promising aspects but there is still no universally accepted way of how this should be performed. One way consists of measuring the distance reached by the regurgitant jet flow imaged from the mitral orifice into the left atrium [41, p. 55]. This will certainly overestimate such regurgitations which have a narrow configuration but reach the posterior atrial wall, as shown in Fig. 6.45b, when compared to others that fill the left atrium in its whole transverse axis, as shown in Fig. 6.45c. In very severe mitral regurgitations with considerable increase in left atrial (and pulmonary) pressure values, however, the systolic transmitral pressure difference may become relatively small, thereby not allowing the regurgitant flow to reach high velocities and much turbulence [86]. In such cases it may become difficult to visualize the incompetence, as can be seen in Fig. 6.46 and 6.49. In these cases the convective acceleration of flow velocities in the left ventricle towards the leak in the mitral valve is a very useful sign (Figs. 6.46, 6.49).

Another way can be adopted from the flow mapping technique using single gate 2D Doppler echocardiography [1, 47]. These investigations have to be performed using the standardized views i.e. as proposed by the American Society of Echocardiography [20]. However, regurgitant flows do not obey these standardizing rules but may take place in a variety of planes which are unpredictable from the conventional 2D image. Such examples are shown in Figs. 6.46 and 6.49. Therefore, the single gate 2D Doppler mapping technique is not able to detect the maximal extension of the regurgitant flow field in every case. Moreover, the standards against which the findings of CBFI are to be compared do not offer absolute parameters. Cineangiocardiography, as the most important method, offers findings which are merely semiquantitative in clinical routine and are liable to interpretational errors. Its semiquantitative approach is based on the time-dependent accumulation of contrast medium in the left atrium during one or more systoles. The approach of CBFI is completely different in that it uses the extension of the regurgitant flow field in one frame as the parameter for grading the severity without accounting for heart rate or other time-dependent factors which also influence the amount of regurgitant volume.

Pitfalls in the diagnosis of mitral valve incompetence may be due to the selection of inappropriate imaging planes. It is our experience that such difficulties arise particularly in severe mitral regurgitation. The example shown in Fig. 6.49 demonstrates the findings in such a severe form. In the apical left-sided two-chamber view (Fig. 6.49) no typical regurgitant flow pattern is detectable other than some low-velocity eddies. It was, however, possible to detect the regurgitant flow by choosing an unusual imaging plane by tilting the transducer from the parasternal long axis towards the right ventricle.

6.4.3 Mitral Valve Prolapse. Mitral valve prolapse may lead to mitral incompetence. In most cases regurgitation starts in mid-to-late systole by prolapse of one or both leaflets into the left atrium. Fig. 6.50 shows the typical time course of late systolic regurgitation in mild incompetence, the 2D insert demonstrates a considerable bulging of the anterior mitral leaflet backwards into the left atrium. The regurgitant jet originates behind the bulge. A more pronounced case of incompetence in mitral valve prolapse is shown in Fig. 6.51 in a young man with Marfan's syndrome. The 2D image displays the thickened mitral valve leaflets which prolapse slightly be-

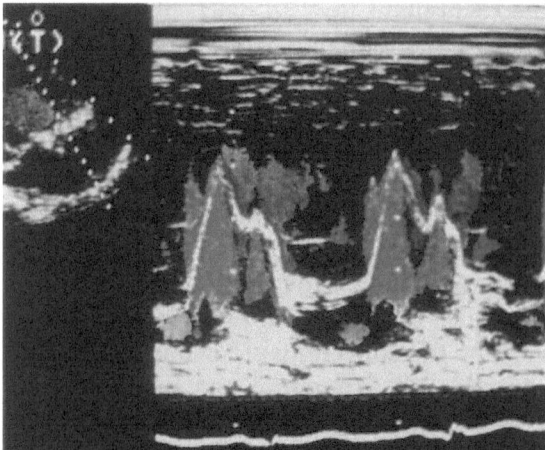

Fig. 6.50 Mitral regurgitation occurring in late systole (*turquoise spot* behind the mitral closure line in the M/Q-mode) caused by mitral valve prolapse (RBG2). In the 2D CBFI insert *(upper left)* a bulging of the anterior mitral leaflet can be seen as well as the hammocking of the mtiral valve closure line in the M/Q-mode

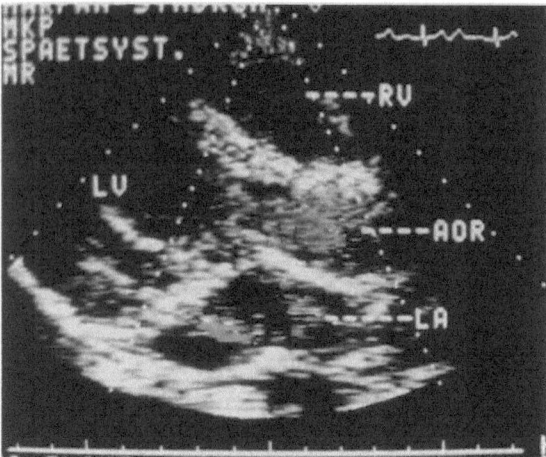

Fig. 6.51 Mitral regurgitation, caused by mitral valve prolapse in Marfan's syndrome (RBG2). A small jet of regurgitant flow can be seen behind the mitral valve commissure in the left atrium *(LA)* together with normal outflow into the aortic root *(AOR)*

hind the plane of the mitral anulus at the end of systole. The incompetence at the coaptation of the anterior and posterior leaflets is clearly visible and is possibly caused by the "myxomatous proliferation" of the valve [46]. Regurgitation started at mid-systole. Estimation of severity from the extension of the regurgitant flow field has to take into account that regurgitation is not holosystolic in these patients.

6.4.4 Mitral Valve Abnormalities in Combination with Other Heart Disease.
Mitral valve disease in combination with other heart disease may occur as mitral regurgitation for instance in *hypertrophic obstructive cardiomyopathy*, as shown in Fig. 6.52. It occurs simultaneously with subaortic obstruction caused by systolic anterior motion (SAM) of the anterior mitral leaflet. This may retract the leaflet from its coaptation with the posterior leaflet and may lead to mitral regurgitation. The theory is enforced by the fact

Fig. 6.52 Mitral regurgitation in hypertrophic obstructive cardiomyopathy, parasternal long axis view (RBG2). Left ventricular outflow tract obstruction is imaged by color aliasing between anterior mitral leaflet and interventricular septum. See text for more details

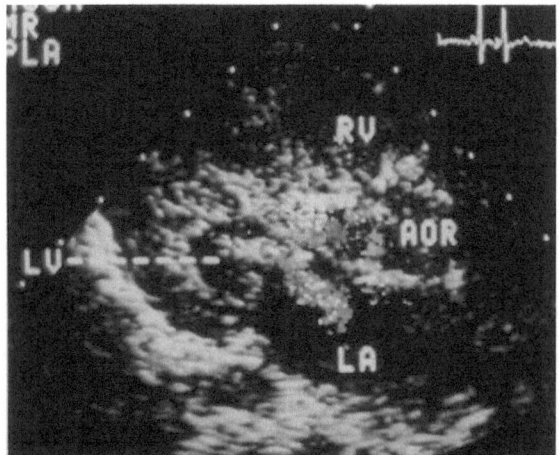

Fig. 6.53 Mitral regurgitation of moderate degree coexisting with tricuspid regurgitation after acute rheumatic fever, apical four-chamber view (RBG2). Mitral incompetence seems to be more severe than tricuspid insufficiency

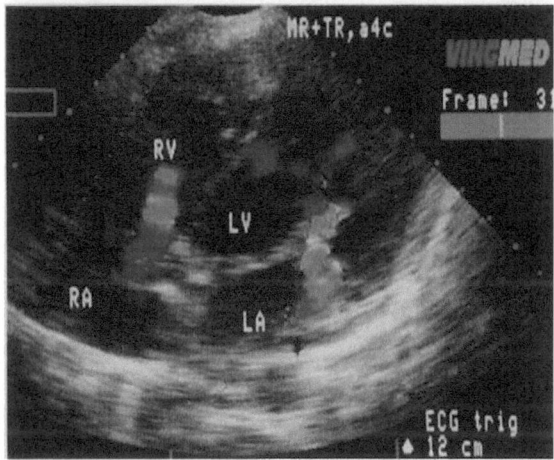

that diminishing SAM by medical treatment can abolish mitral regurgitation, as shown in Fig. 6.64b, c (p. 94).

In *dilative cardiomyopathy* mitral incompetence is caused by the dilatation of the left ventricular cavity with subsequent enlargement of the mitral valve anulus. This may cause a dehiscence of the mitral commissures which will lead to mitral regurgitation, as shown in Fig. 6.45a (p. 80).

Mitral and tricuspid regurgitation often coexist together, in many cases mitral valvular heart disease is the primary lesion. In Fig. 6.53 the incompetence of both valves is caused by rheumatic fever.

In *endocardial cushion defect* malformations of the atrioventricular valves occur together with ASDs and VSDs. These malformations include clefts, especially of the mitral leaflet, which lead to mitral regurgitation (Fig. 6.54) and atypical insertion of the anterior leaflet of the mitral valve causing an atypical diastolic opening motion [87].

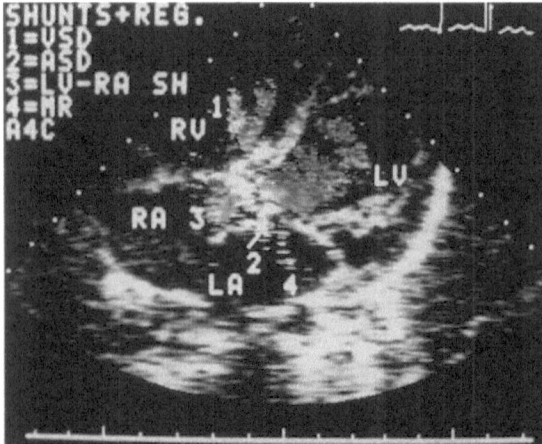

Fig. 6.54 Pathological flow conditions in endocardial cushion defect of the intermediate type (RBG2). Systolic frame of pathological flow conditions, apical four-chamber view (see also Fig. 6.28 b). Slight mitral regurgitation *(4)* is shown together with left ventricular-right atrial shunt *(3)* and left-to-right shunt across the atrial *(2)* and ventricular septal defects *(1)*

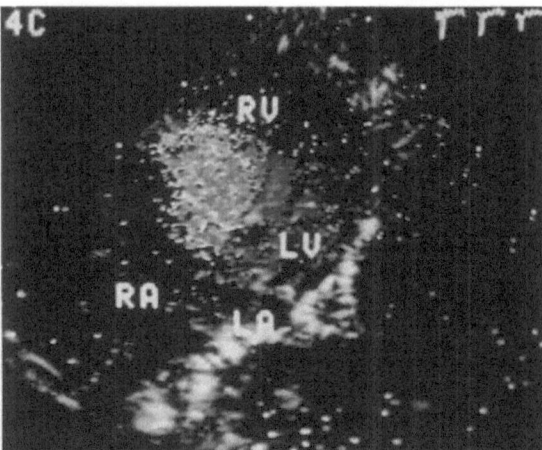

Fig. 6.55 Diastolic atrioventricular valve flow in mitral valve atresia in hypoplastic left heart syndrome, apical four-chamber view (RBG2). The tricuspid valve is wide open allowing inflow from the right atrium *(RA)* into right ventricle *(RV),* colored *red-orange.* The mitral valve is completely atretic, not allowing any diastolic flow from the hypoplastic left atrium *(LA)* into the diminutive left ventricle *(LV)*

Mitral atresia is always combined with additional, usually severe, cardiac malformations. Fig. 6.55 shows an example in which mitral atresia is accompanied by hypoplasia of the left atrium, the left ventricle and the aortic valve (not shown here); it forms a part of the so-called *hypoplastic left-heart syndrome.*

6.5 Abnormalities of the Left Ventricular Outflow and the Aorta

The left ventricular outflow tract may be considered to extend from the free edges of the anterior mitral leaflet down to the bifurcation of the abdominal aorta [78]. There are therefore several levels at which structural abnormalities may cause blood flow abnormalities, i.e., the aortic valve and the aortic root, the subaortic area, or the region of the isthmus.

6.5.1 Aortic Stenosis. Aortic valve stenosis is the most common lesion causing flow abnormalities in the left ventricular outflow. It is characterized by the appearance of pathologically high velocities leading to turbulence but appearing at correct timing. Fig. 6.56 shows the systolic doming of the aortic valve in mild aortic stenosis causing a decrease of outflow diameter from 20 mm to 12 mm at the valve level. Flow velocities can be seen to accelerate inside the dome towards the orifice above which color aliasing indicates the formation of the jet. Fig. 6.57 demonstrates the morphological and rheological findings in a more severe form. The valve leaflets are severely restricted in their motion and appear like a membrane across the aortic orifice. Systolic outflow accelerates 5 mm proximal to the stenotic valve and rapidly reaches high velocities within the stenotic valve orifice. This is recognizable from the peculiar pattern of aliasing that takes place from the away-direction in the left ventricle to the towards-direction of the jet in the aortic root without color change. The jet (turquoise) is directed towards the anterior wall of the aortic root and is surrounded by a layer of lower flow velocities representing parajet phenomena. Their velocities are below the Nyquist limit of pulsed sampling and are therefore imaged in red-yellow. The areas of lower velocities represent the shear lay-

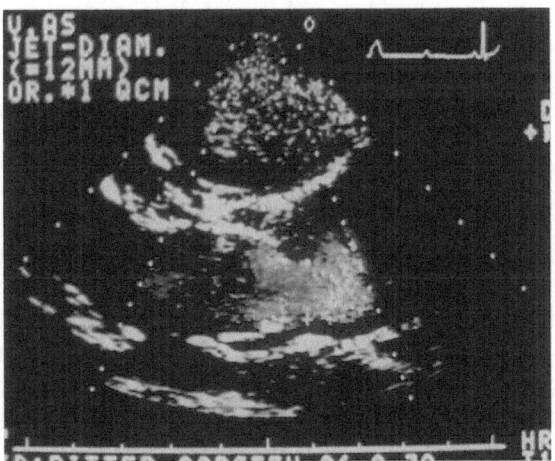

Fig. 6.56 Mild aortic valve stenosis showing typical systolic doming of aortic valves causing outflow disturbances at the valve orifice and in the ascending aorta. See text for more details

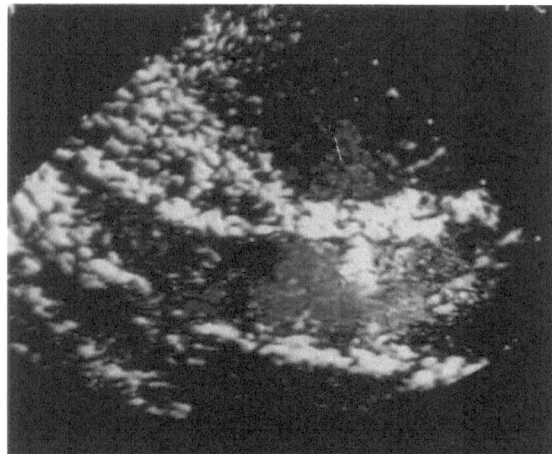

a

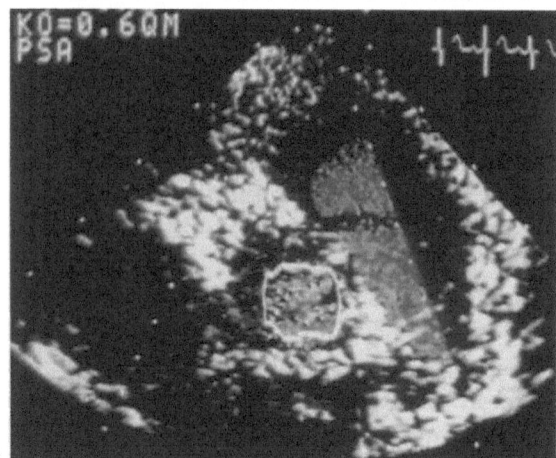

b

Fig. 6.57 a, b Severe aortic stenosis with nearly immobile aortic valves and considerable septal hypertrophy.
a Systolic jet in aortic stenosis, parasternal long axis view (RBG2). CBFI reveals acceleration of left ventricular outflow velocities towards the stenotic orifice passing it as a narrow-based jet. See text for more details

b Same jet-like flow in aortic stenosis as in **a**, image in the parasternal short axis view. The physiological outflow into pulmonary artery is displayed in *blue* (incompletely because of color sector limitation)

ers along and around the jet. It is evident from Fig. 6.57a that the high-velocity core of the jet becomes narrower with increasing distance from the valve orifice, as predicted by the laws of hydrodynamics [45]. The stenotic jet can also be visualized in the ascending aorta from the suprasternal position, as shown in Fig. 6.58. Here the jet is represented by the turquoise area surrounded by the red-yellow normal outflow in the ascending aorta, where it can be reached easily by the continuous Doppler investigation.

The flow phenomena of aortic stenosis can also be imaged in the short axis view, as shown in Fig. 6.57b. From this it is evident that the area of outflowing blood is significantly reduced when compared with normal findings (see Fig. 5.8, p. 32). This is, however, not a true measure of the aortic orifice like in mitral stenosis (see p. 77) because the high jet velocities in aortic stenosis induce the build-up of pronounced parajet phenomena, as shown in Fig. 6.57a. Somtimes the core of the jet can be distinguished

Fig. 6.58 Jet of aortic stenosis imaged by aliasing within the normal systolic towards-flow in the ascending aorta from the suprasternal position. The jet is represented by the *turquoise area* surrounded by *red-yellow* normal outflow. See text for more details

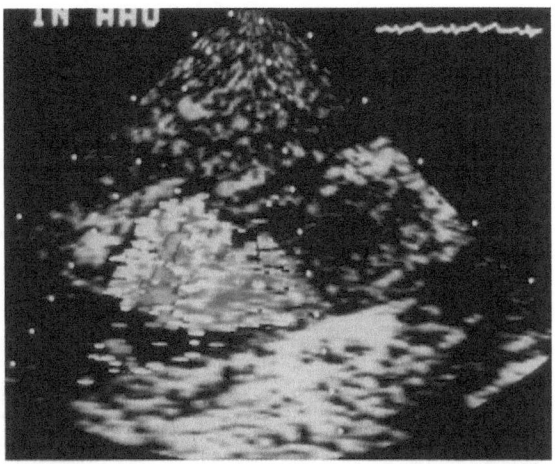

from the parajet flow, as shown in Fig. 6.59 b. In such cases CBFI may help to define the valve opening area more precisely than 2D echocardiography, as can be seen from Fig. 6.59.

In *critical valvular aortic stenosis* of the newborn, the volume flow rate delivered through the highly stenotic aortic valve orifice into the aorta is not sufficient to meet the demands of the body. As long as the ductus arteriosus is patent, it will make up for this deficit by shunting pulmonary arterial blood into the aorta. This will lead to retrograde perfusion of all or parts of the aortic arch. Fig. 6.60 shows a CBFI image of the aorta, which has a diameter of about 5 mm, from the suprasternal position in critical aortic stenosis. It demonstrates that most of the ascending aorta is perfused in a retrograde fashion during systole, as can be seen from the blue coloration (compare Fig. 4.4, p. 24). The jet flow through the highly narrowed aortic orifice fills only parts of the aortic root with normal antegrade flow (yellow-red).

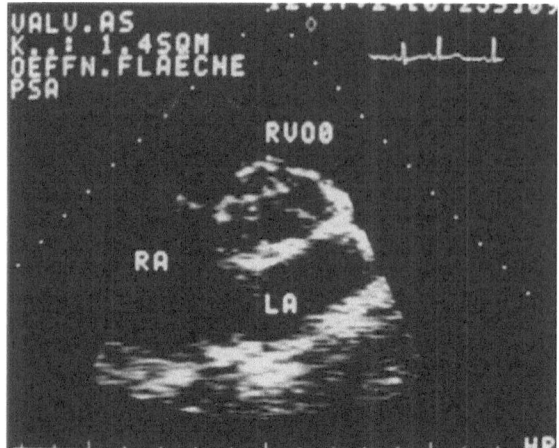

a

Fig. 6.59 a, b Moderately severe aortic stenosis in the parasternal short axis view.
a The 2D image shows incomplete opening of aortic valves in early systole

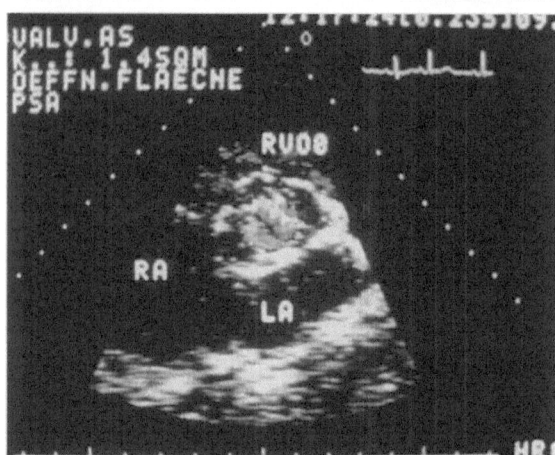

b

b Superposition of CBFI shows clearly the core of the jet *(turquoise)* together with some eddy formation *(orange-yellow)*

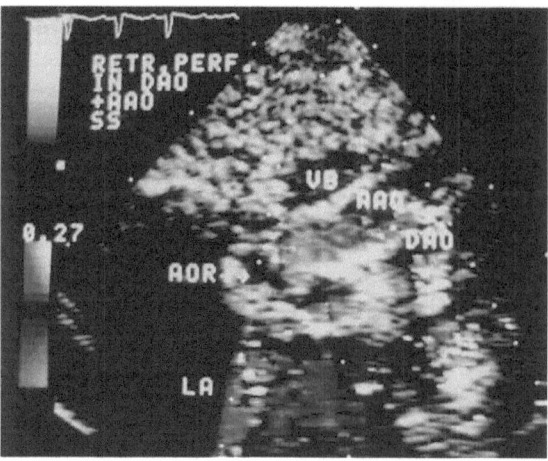

Fig. 6.60 Critical aortic stenosis in a neonate, visualized from the suprasternal position. CBFI (RBG2) demonstrates the retrograde perfusion of most of the ascending aorta *(AAO) (blue)* while the normal anterograde flow is limited to the aortic root *(yellow-red)*. Blood passing through the severely stenosed aortic valve is shown in *yellow-turquoise* mosaic pattern

Fig. 6.61 a, b Aortic valve atresia in hypoplastic left heart syndrome in a neonate, imaged from the suprasternal position.
a The hypoplastic ascending aorta *(AAO)* can be seen to cross the right pulmonic artery *(RPA)*

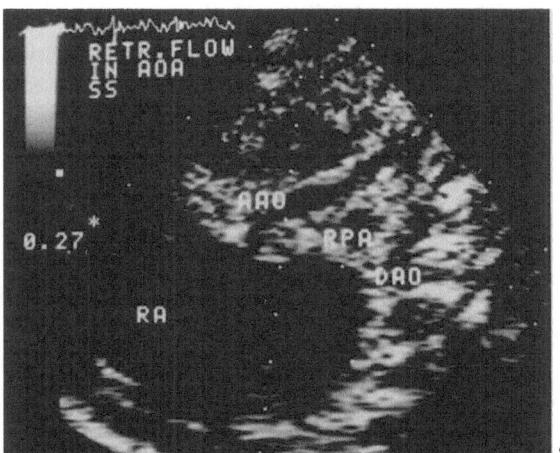

b Superposition of CBFI proves that the whole proximal aorta is perfused in a retrograde fashion from the ductal orifice to the aortic root. RB1 color display has been chosen to show clearly the low velocities of blood flow in the ascending aorta which only serves the coronary perfusion

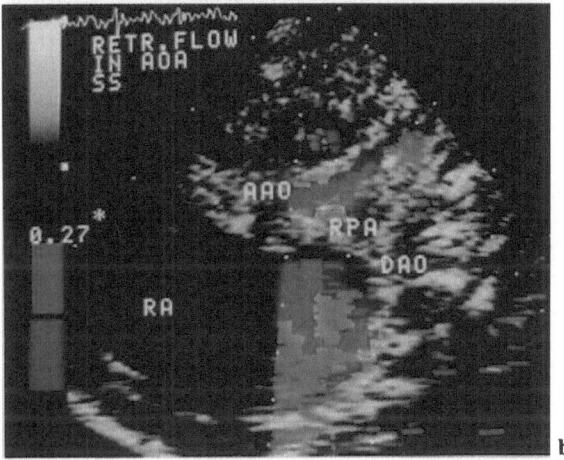

6.5.2 Aortic Valve Atresia. Aortic valve atresia is a condition in which an imperforate aortic valve does not allow any normal outflow from the left ventricular cavity into the aortic root. Usually, the ascending aorta and the proximal arch are severely hypoplastic. This condition is usually found in association with severe mitral stenosis or mitral valve atresia (see section 6.4.6) and forms, together with hypoplasia of the left atrium and left ventricle, the so-called *hypoplastic left-heart syndrome*. Fig. 6.61a demonstrates the hypoplasia of the ascending aorta and the proximal aortic arch in aortic atresia, the diameter of the ascending aorta is about 3 mm. Superposition of CBFI in Fig. 6.61b proves the diagnosis by showing a retrograde perfusion of the proximal aorta down to the aortic root (red in the descending aorta and blue in the ascending aorta) which is maintained by right-to-left shunt across a PDA and serves only the perfusion of the coronary circulation.

Diagnostic pitfalls in aortic stenosis may occur as false negative results if several of the standardized views are not used. In our experience it is not easy, and sometimes even impossible, to visualize the jet. However, any color change at the level of the aortic valve is highly suggestive of valvular stenosis.

6.5.3 Subaortic Stenosis. Subaortic stenosis is caused either by a fixed anatomical or by a functional alteration in the left ventricular outflow tract (LVO). In the first case, the underlying cause may be a discrete membrane (Fig. 6.62 a) or a muscular ridge located in the LVO beneath the aortic leaflets or a funnel-shaped narrowing of the LVO. The typical example of a *functional* outflow obstruction is found in hypertrophic obstructive cardiomyopathy (HOCM), which has also been called "idiopathic hypertrophic subaortic stenosis" (IHSS) and will be referred to later in this chapter.

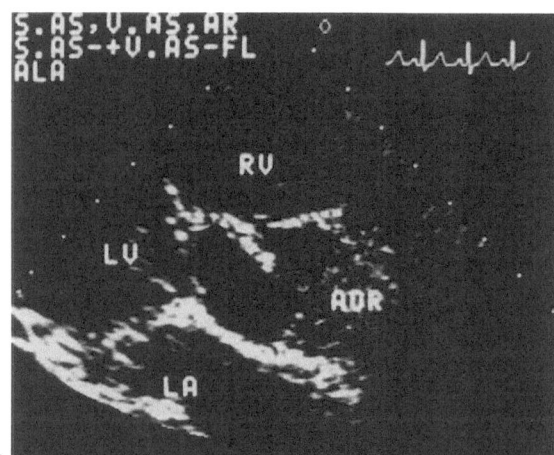

Fig. 6.62 a, b Discrete subaortic stenosis caused by a membrane-like structure with a central hole encircling the left venzricular outflow tract immediately below the aortic valve. Parasternal long axis view, systolic frame.

a The 2D image shows the membrane proximal to the incomplete systolic opening of the right coronary cusp

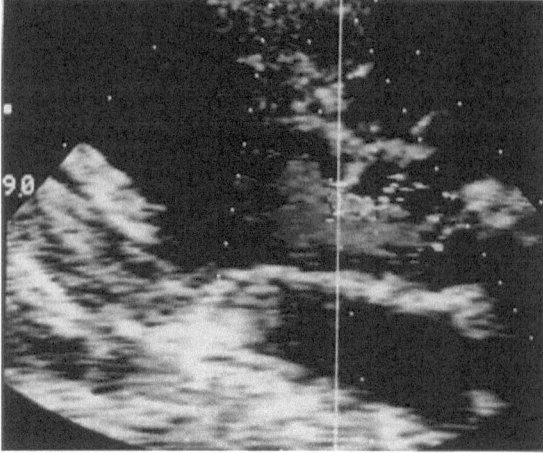

b CBFI shows turbulence, aliasing and eddy formation at and distal to the stenotic membrane which are extending into the aorta

Fig. 6.63 M/Q-mode of aortic root (RBG2). It can be seen that flow is normal only in the very early systole when the aortic valve opens completely for a short period of time. See text for more details

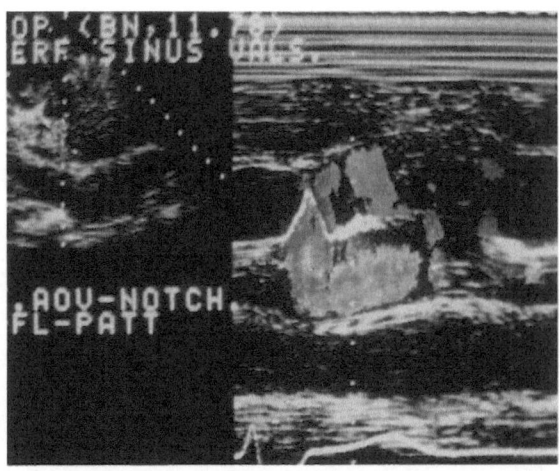

In both conditions there is systolic turbulence in the LVO proximal to the aortic valve. In *discrete subaortic stenosis,* flow disturbances start at the membrane and extend into the aortic root, thereby causing the typical mid-systolic notching of the right coronary cusp [9]. In Fig. 6.62 both pictures show the same morphology but flow information is absent in Fig. 6.62 a. Considerable narrowing of the outflow tract is caused by a fibrous ridge protruding from the interventricular septum into the outflow cavity. The right coronary cusp of the aortic valve is seen in a semiclosed position in mid-systole. Adding flow information to the picture (Fig. 6.62 b) makes it clear that the subaortic membrane is causing flow disturbances which extend beyond the valve into the aortic root.

Fig. 6.63 shows the blood flow pattern in the aortic valve orifice itself. The RBG2 color code has been chosen and normal systolic flow is imaged in yellow-red. In the early part of systole, preclosure of the right coronary cusp can be seen and is accompanied by a short phase of backflow inside the orifice near the commissure. Coarse fluttering of the valve is indicated by additional small backflow areas during the later part of systole. The area between the aortic wall and the valve is occupied by blood which is flowing away from the transducer. This indicates that the Venturi effect is responsible for the preclosure of the aortic right coronary cusp, as had already been suspected earlier [13].

Hypertrophic obstructive cardiomyopathy causes outflow stenosis which may involve different parts of the mitral valve apparatus, i.e., the anterior or posterior leaflet or the chordae tendineae [69] by causing, them to move anteriorly in systole (systolic anterior motion – SAM). In Fig. 6.64 a late systolic frame of a patient with HOCM and Friedreich's ataxia is shown, SAM of the auterior mitral leaflet is clearly visible protruding into the outflow tract. Superposition of CBFI (Fig. 6.64 b) shows that severe flow dis-

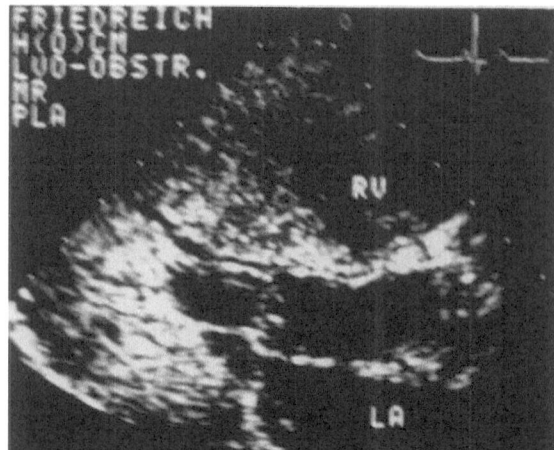

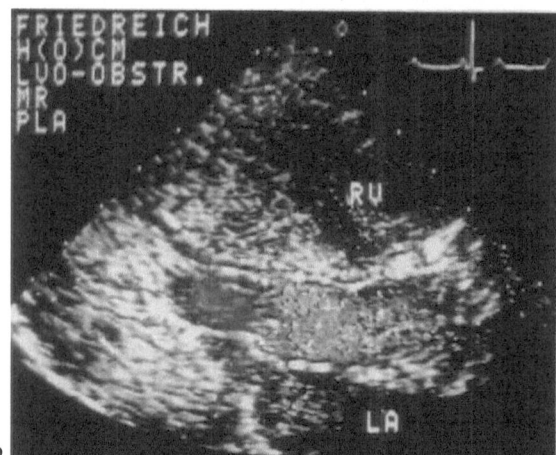

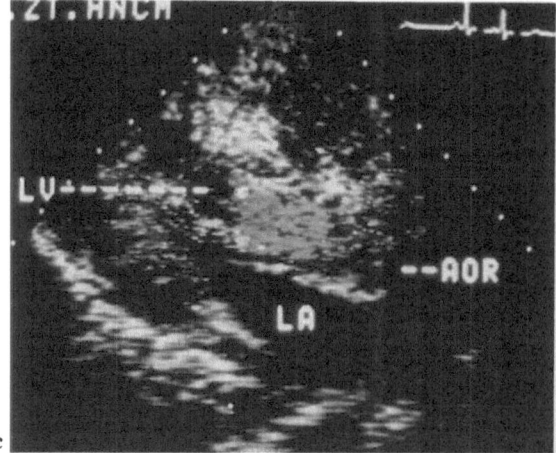

Fig. 6.64a–c Left ventricular outflow tract stenosis in hypertrophic obstructive cardiomyopathy.
a Systolic 2D image of the left ventricular outflow tract in the parasternal long axis view showing systolic anterior motion (SAM) of the chordae at the tip of the anterior mitral leaflet

b Superposition of CBFI shows the origin of flow disturbances *(mosaic coloration)* at the SAM extending distally into the outflow tract and across the aortic valve. There is also mitral incompetence indicated by *color mosaic* in the left atrium *(LA)*

c Flow disturbances in the left ventricular outflow tract have disappeared 6 months later under treatment with a beta-blocking agent as indicated by the homogeneous *blue coloration*. Mitral regurgitation has subsided as well

Fig. 6.65 M/Q-mode in hypertrophic obstructive cardiomyopathy shows that SAM is causing turbulence from mid-systole on between the anterior leaflet of the mitral valve and the interventricular septum. Additionally, mitral incompetence can be seen to occur in diastole indicated by the *blue area* at the mitral closure line

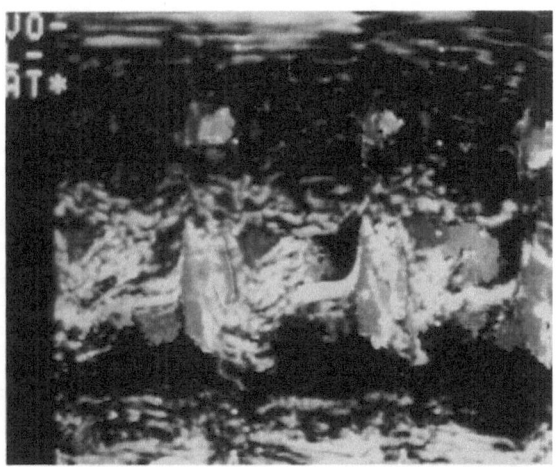

turbance – imaged as a mosaic flow pattern – is caused by the SAM in the subaortic region. Additionally, mitral incompetence, which often accompanies HOCM, is seen to cause regurgitation into the left atrium (see also Fig. 6.65). Obstruction in HOCM is dynamic and may subside during treatment. This is shown in Fig. 6.64 c which was taken from the same patient 6 months later under treatment with a beta-blocking agent. There is no longer any SAM and blood is flowing undisturbed into the aortic root. Mitral regurgitation has also subsided indicating that it had been caused by traction of the mitral leaflet into the outflow tract and is reversible if the SAM disappears.

6.5.4 Coarctation of the Aorta. Coarctation of the aorta can often be visualized by 2D echocardiography [68, 79]. It is, however, our experience that complete visualization is frequently not possible [50]. In such instances CBFI may help to overcome these limitations. In Fig. 6.66 the aortic arch is visualized from the suprasternal position where a shelf-like constriction is found protruding into the lumen of the proximal part of the descending aorta (Fig. 6.66 a). There is poststenotic dilatation as would be expected in simple coarctation. Superposition of CBFI (Fig. 6.66 b) shows that flow acceleration takes place immediately proximal to and at the stenotic shelf as indicated by aliasing from blue to orange-yellow, and extends as a jet into the poststenotic dilatation.

Flow patterns in the *descending aorta* change from the normal systolic pulsating pattern (Fig. 6.67 a) to a continuously systolic-diastolic streaming pattern (Fig. 6.67 b) owing to the prolonged passage of blood through the stenotic isthmus and the collateral vessels.

Infantile preductal coarctation can be visualized directly using CBFI (Fig. 6.68) as can the vitally important right-to-left shunt across the PDA

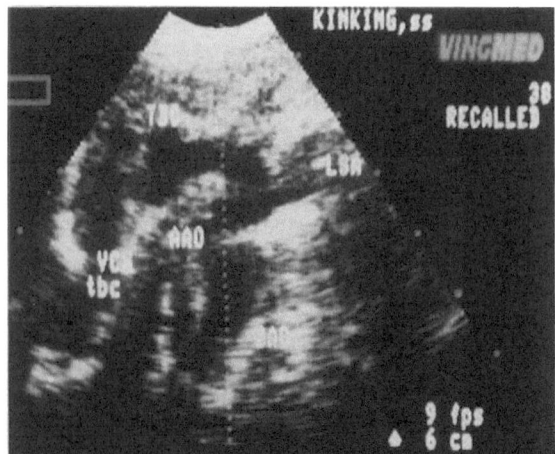

a

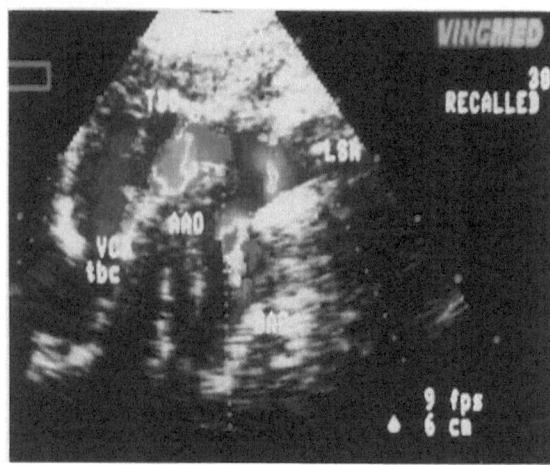

b

Fig. 6.66 a, b Stenotic narrowing in aortic coarctation. Long axis view of the aortic arch from the suprasternal position.
a A shelf-like structure can be seen protruding into the proximal part of the descending aorta *(DAO)* which is dilated more distally

b Superposition of CBFI shows aliasing and flow disturbances (green-yellow) at the stenotic area of the coarctation caused by convective acceleration and extending below the narrowing (RBG2)

into the descending aorta (see Fig. 6.38 a, p. 75). In many infants the ductal patency is dependent on prostaglandin E, thus the effectivity of its application is directly visible. In most cases a VSD is also present and shows a bidirectional shunt pattern (see Fig. 6.16 b, p. 57). Additionally, we have always found an incomplete foramen ovale with its typical left-to-right shunt pattern. These accompanying hemodynamic findings are very useful diagnostic aids which will quickly lead the investigator to the correct diagnosis.

Diagnostic pitfalls may be caused by the normal parabolic flow profile in the proximal part of the descending aorta which causes color aliasing in the centre (see Fig. 5.9 a, p. 33) and may be mistaken for turbulent flow in coarctation. The absence of a morphological narrowing, however, and the normal flow pattern in the descending aorta will help to avoid this false positive diagnosis.

Fig. 6.67 a, b M/Q-mode and single gate Doppler FFT trace of blood flow in the descending aorta recorded from the subcostal position from where blood flow is directed towards the transducer (RBG2).

a Normal pulsatile systolic flow pattern. Diastolic velocities are below the CBFI threshold

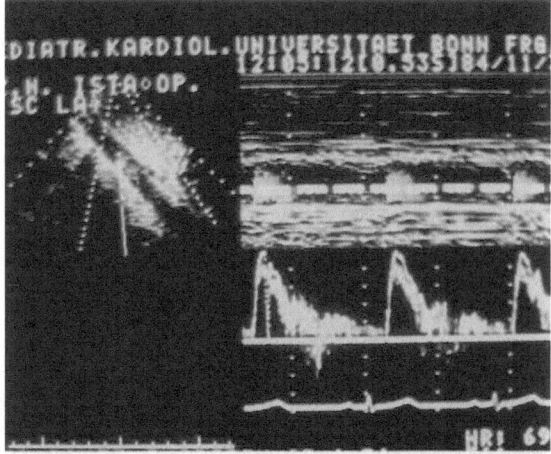

b Almost continuous systolic-diastolic flow in the descending aorta caused by coarctation

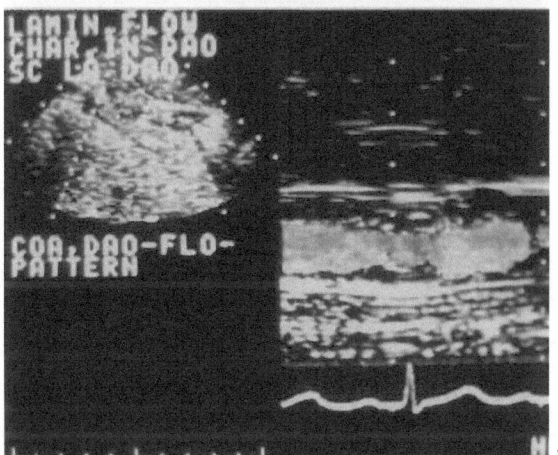

Fig. 6.68 Infantile iuxtaductal coarctation visualized from the suprasternal position (RBG2). The tubular hypoplasia of the distal aortic arch *(aoa)* shows up in *turquoise* as does the wider proximal part of the descending aorta *(DAO)* which is perfused via the PDA (see Fig. 6.38 a)

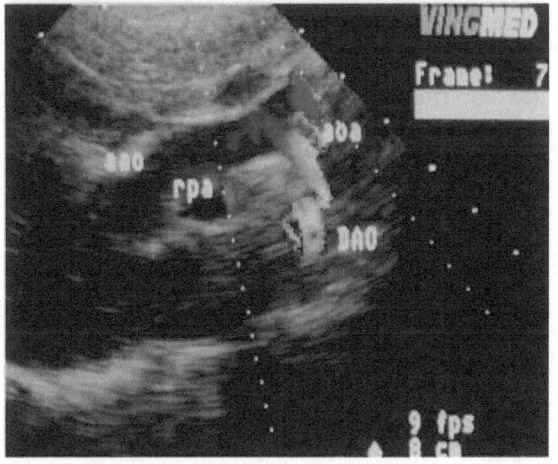

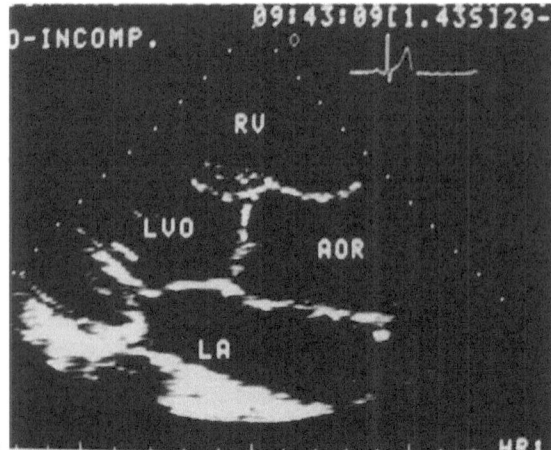

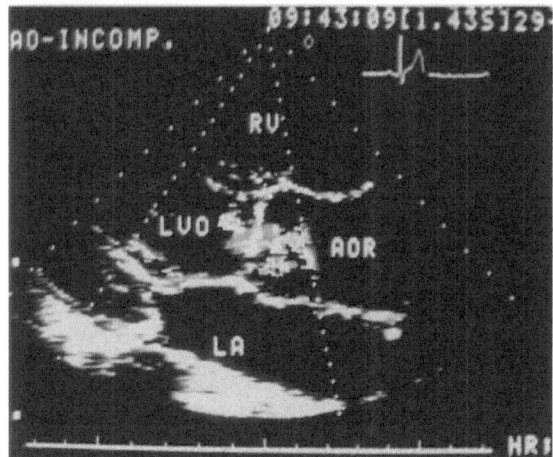

Fig. 6.69 a, b Very slight aortic regurgitation, parasternal long axis view.
a The 2D image of the left ventricular outflow tract *(LVO)* in early diastole and aortic root *(AOR)* does not show any abnormalities

b Superposition of CBFI demonstrates a small jet crossing the aortic valve straight into the outflow tract *(turquoise)*

6.5.5 Aortic Regurgitation. Aortic regurgitation can be diagnosed very reliably by pulsed wave Doppler [75, 77]. The finding of a turbulent diastolic high velocity flow pattern in the left ventricular outflow tract is diagnostic for aortic incompetence; its shape, direction, and distribution are directly imaged by CBFI and represent the regurgitant jet. There are three possible jet directions: the regurgitant flow may splash straight into the outflow tract without reaching its anterior or posterior border (see Fig. 4.5, p. 25, and Fig. 6.69 b); it may run into the posterior direction and bounce against the anterior mitral leaflet (Fig. 6.70), which is most common in aortic incompetence; or it may be directed anteriorly towards the interventricular septum (Fig. 6.71).

Indirect signs of these different jet routes cause the well-known echocardiographic signs of fine diastolic fluttering of the anterior mitral leaflet or of the interventricular septum [21, 16]. The time course of this fluttering

Fig. 6.70 Aortic regurgitation visualized in the parasternal long axis view (RBG2). The regurgitant jet *(turquoise)* can be seen to splash against the middle part of the anterior mitral valve leaflet hereby bulging it into the left atrium *(LA)*

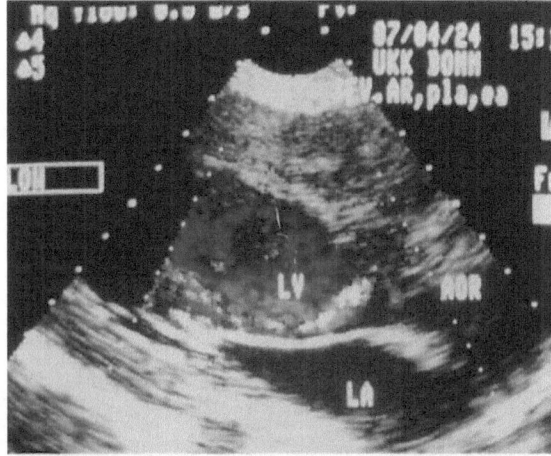

Fig. 6.71 Mild aortic incompetence in the parasternal long axis view (RBG2). The jet *(red-turquoise)* is directed towards the interventricular septum, the anterior mitral valve leaflet is just starting to open (indicated by *red coloration*)

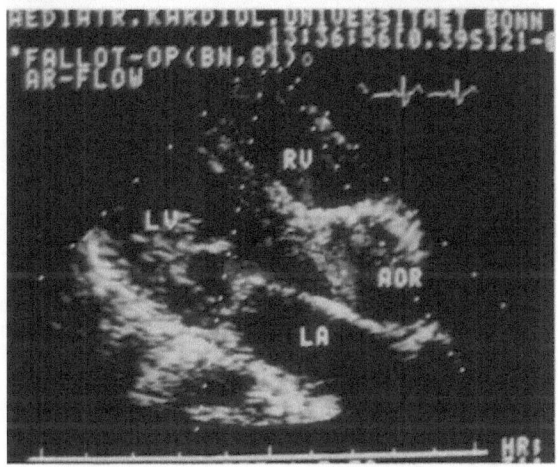

can be shown using the M/Q-mode (Fig. 6.72 a). Less frequently, diastolic fluttering of the aortic valve is observed [12], the corresponding finding in the M/Q-mode is shown in Fig. 6.72 b. There are several other echocardiographic planes by which the flow phenomena of aortic insufficiency can be imaged. They include the apical four-chamber view (Fig. 6.73), which is usually applicable even in patients who are difficult to investigate, or the different levels of the parasternal short axis view (Fig. 6.74, 6.75). In the short axis view of the great arteries, the diastolic leak in the aortic valve can be imaged thus allowing an accurate identification of the leaking commissure(s) (Fig. 6.74). The cross-sectional area of the jet determined by planimetry has been used to quantify aortic regurgitation [28] as has already been proposed for conventional single gate Doppler [76]. It is important to determine the area at the level of the aortic valve because the jet diameter increases downwards in the left ventricle (Fig. 6.70). The mu-

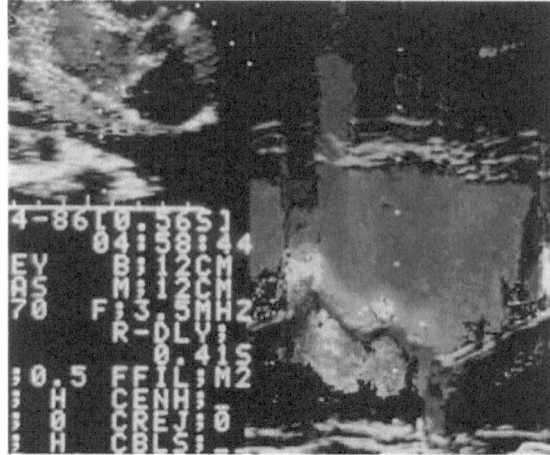

Fig. 6.72 a, b Appearance of aortic regurgitation in the M/Q-mode. **a** Positioning the M/Q-line at the middle of the anterior mitral valve leaflet (as shown in the 2D insert - *upper left*) demonstrates the rebound of the regurgitant jet against the mitral leaflet *(yellow-turquoise)* which causes the well-known mitral flutter

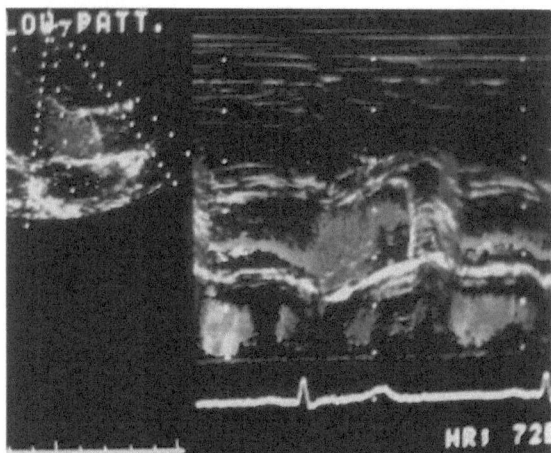

b Positioning the M/Q-line in the distal left ventricular outflow tract (see the 2D insert - *upper left*) shows the regurgitant jet passing through the valve commissures in diastole *(turquoise-yellow)* and the normal systolic outflow, as indicated by the *blue coloration* of the aortic valve "box" in systole

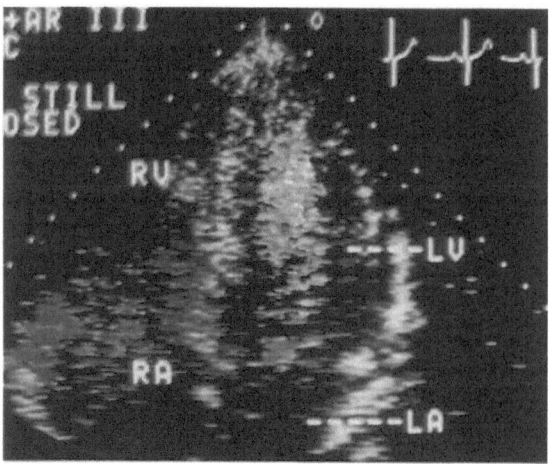

Fig. 6.73 Severe aortic regurgitation in the apical four-chamber view (RBG2). The regurgitant jet *(yellow-turquoise)* extends into the apex of the left ventricle *(LV)* in early diastole, as indicated by the start of the opening movement of the mitral valve

Fig. 6.74 Aortic regurgitation imaged in the parasternal short axis view at the level of the aortic commissures (RBG2). The leak can be seen at the centre of the three commissures *(turquoise-red)*. *R*, right coronary cusp; *L*, left coronary cusp; *N*, noncoronary cusp

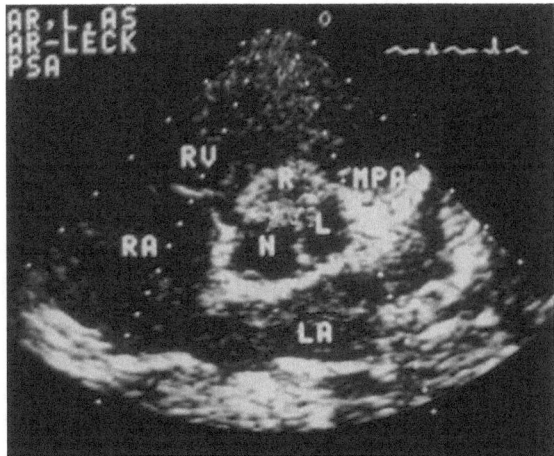

Fig. 6.75 Mutual influence of aortic regurgitation and mitral inflow (RBG2), see also Fig. 6.70. In the parasternal short axis view at the mitral valve level the jet flattens the mitral opening area in moderately severe aortic incompetence. See text for more details

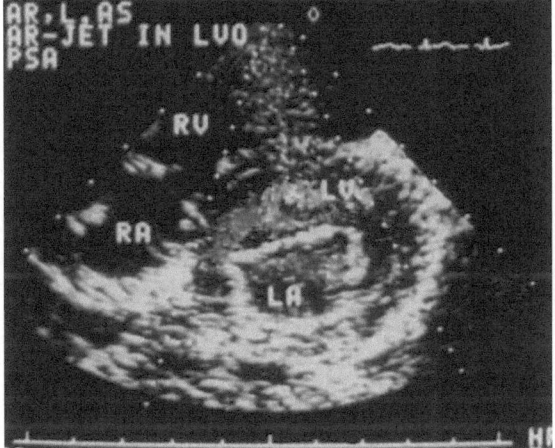

tual interplay between the diastolic filling of the left ventricle through the mitral valve and the regurgitant jet can be studied in detail using CBFI. Fig. 6.70 shows a long axis view of the left ventricle in a patient with mild aortic incompetence. The bouncing of the regurgitant jet against the anterior mitral leaflet causes a bulge back into the left atrium (reversed doming).

In Fig. 6.75 the influence of the regurgitant jet on the opening configuration of the mitral orifice can be observed in a patient with moderately severe incompetence during late diastole (600 ms after R) in the parasternal short axis view at the mitral valve level. The normally semi-oval configuration of the anterior leaflet is flattened causing the phenomenon of "reversed doming" which has been described in the parasternal long axis view (see Fig. 6.70) [58]. Inflowing blood from the left atrium (yellow-orange near the septum) has to give way to the regurgitant flow (mosaic pattern in turquoise).

For *semiquantification* of aortic incompetence, several measurement parameters of the regurgitating jet have been proposed. One proposal uses the depth of the jet from the aortic valve into the left ventricle [42]. This has been adopted from the mapping technique using the conventional single gate 2D Doppler method [72]. Another approach has already been mentioned in which the cross-sectional jet area at the level of the aortic valve has been used [28]. A third proposal is to determine the regurgitant volume by biplane Simpson's rule from the planimetered area of the jet in the apical two- and five-chamber views [6]. It has, however, not been mentioned by the authors how regurgitant volume flow can be obtained from these measurements. The fourth possibility is the determination of the ratio of jet width over left ventricular outflow tract width which has been reported to give the best correlation with angiocardiographic grading in one comparative study [8].

Before the results of different studies can be compared there has to be made an agreement on the diastolic timing of jet evaluation since we have discussed above that there is mutual interference between the configuration of the regurgitant jet and the mitral valve orifice. In our opinion, the most suitable moment is the period of isovolumetric relaxation during which the mitral valve is still closed (see Figs. 6.69 b–6.71, p. 98, 99, 6.73, p. 100). The phase of isovolumetric contraction may be less appropriate because at this time the pressure difference between the aorta and the left ventricle is smaller and prohibits the full development of the jet.

Various grades of severity of aortic incompetence are shown in the figures of this chapter at different points of the cardiac cycle. A very mild regurgitation is imaged in Fig. 6.69 b (p. 98) at the end of diastole. Both the mitral and aortic valves are in a closed position, a small regurgitant jet (yellow) is entering the left ventricular outflow tract. Fig. 6.70 (p. 99) shows a moderately severe aortic incompetence (grade 3 according to Sellers [63] at early diastole, the mitral valve leaflets are both in a nearly closed position. The mosaic pattern of regurgitation extends down to the level of the papillary muscles. In Fig. 6.76 severe aortic regurgitation is imaged in late diastole. A considerable part of the left ventricular cavity is still filled by the regurgitation volume of aortic incompetence.

Combined aortic valve disease is relatively common in congenitally malformed aortic valves. Fig. 6.77 shows aortic stenosis (upper frame) and mild regurgitation (lower frame) in such a condition. The aortic valve is morphologically thickened and immobile in systole (see Fig. 6.57, p. 88), in diastole a small-based jet can be seen extending into the left ventricular outflow tract over only a short distance.

Diagnostic pitfalls may occur if the timing of diastolic flow abnormalities is not observed carefully [81]. Fig. 6.78 shows an example in which a strange color phenomenon in the left ventricular outflow tract was misin-

Fig. 6.76 Severe aortic regurgitation in late diastole (RBG2). The left ventricular cavity is filled almost completely by the regurgitant blood

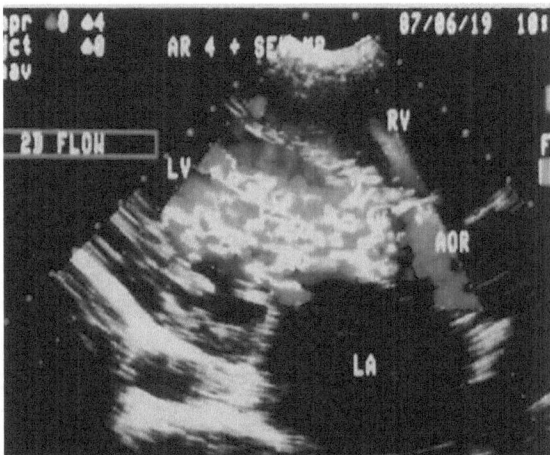

Fig. 6.77 Congenital aortic stenosis *(upper frame)* and incompetence *(lower frame)* in a bicuspid aortic valve, parasternal long axis view (RBG2). The *upper frame* is the same as in Fig. 6.57a. See text for more details

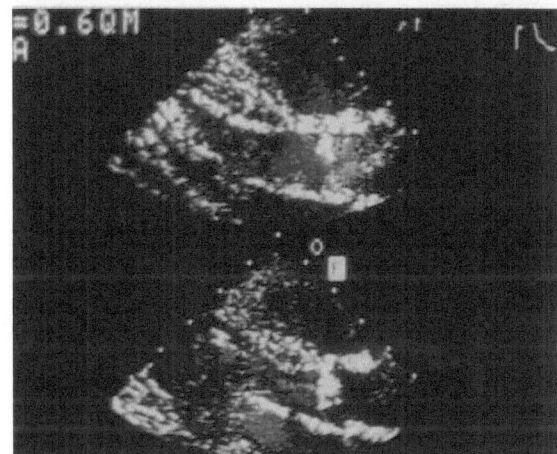

Fig. 6.78 False-positive finding of aortic regurgitation, parasternal long axis view, early diastole (RBG2). The *seven asterisks* mark the red-yellow area which appeared in early systole in the left ventricular outflow tract and represents an artefact which may have been caused by the mirroring of transmitral inflow at the interventricular septum (see p. 14)

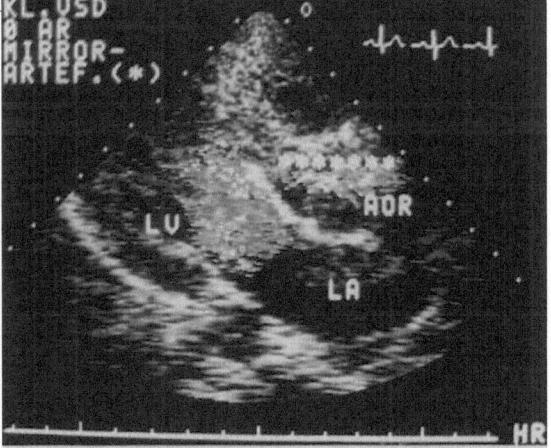

terpreted as aortic regurgitation. More exact observation of timing would have revealed that this phenomenon only appeared in early diastole. It is therefore unlikely that it could have been caused by aortic incompetence.

6.5.6 Aortic Abnormalities in Complex Heart Disease. Aortic valve disease, which is always combined with additional cardiac malformations, is represented by aortic valve atresia. Together with mitral valve atresia it forms the *hypoplastic left heart syndrome* which has been referred to earlier (see p. 91). In 5% of *VSDs* of either the supracristal or the infracristal type, *aortic valve incompetence* is found in addition [73]. In Fig. 6.79 the regurgitant jet can be seen to run along the ventricular septum into the left ventricle as well as to enter the right ventricle through the infracristal defect.

Aortic regurgitation may also be found in *conotruncal malformations* like truncus arteriosus or tetralogy of Fallot [27]. In Fig. 6.80 severe incompetence is shown in truncus arteriosus caused by a quadruspid truncal

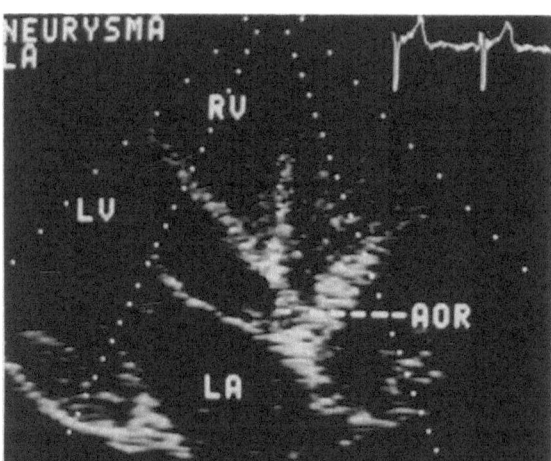

Fig. 6.79 Aortic regurgitation in combination with a infracristal ventricular septal defect, apical long axis view (RBG2). The regurgitant jet can be seen to run along the interventricular septum *(red-yellow)* as well as to enter the right ventricle *(RV)* through the defect *(turquoise-yellow)*

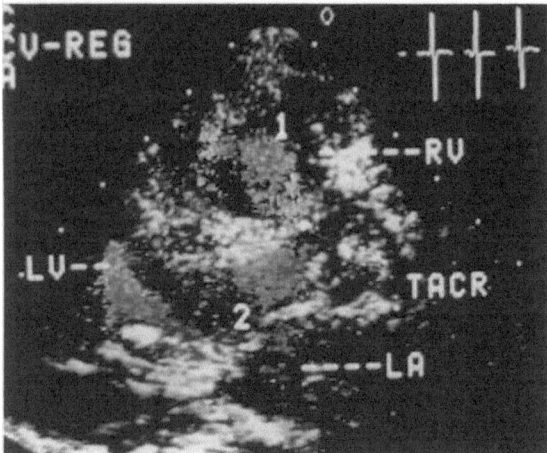

Fig. 6.80 Diastolic frame of truncus arteriosus in a low parasternal long axis view (RBG2). Severe incompetence of the quadricuspid truncal valve causes diastolic backflow into the right *(red-yellow, 1)* and left ventricles *(blue, 2)*. Additionally, blood is entering the left ventricle across the mitral valve *(red yellow)*. TACR - root of the truncus arteriosus

valve. Regurgitant blood entering the right ventricle is imaged in yellow-red, blood entering the left ventricle is shown in blue-cyan.

6.6 Abnormalities of the Right Ventricular Inflow

Abnormalities of the right ventricular inflow tract have a similar appearance in CBFI to those of the left side. Nevertheless, there are some striking differences which will be pointed out on the following pages.

6.6.1 Tricuspid Stenosis. Tricuspid stenosis is a rare organic disease which causes diastolic flow disturbances by increased inflow velocities into the right ventricle. Fig. 6.81 demonstrates right ventricular inflow disturbances in congenital tricuspid stenosis. Even slight narrowing of the tricuspid orifice shows up easily in CBFI, as can be seen in Fig. 6.82 taken in a neonate. The inflow area of the right side is clearly brighter than that of the

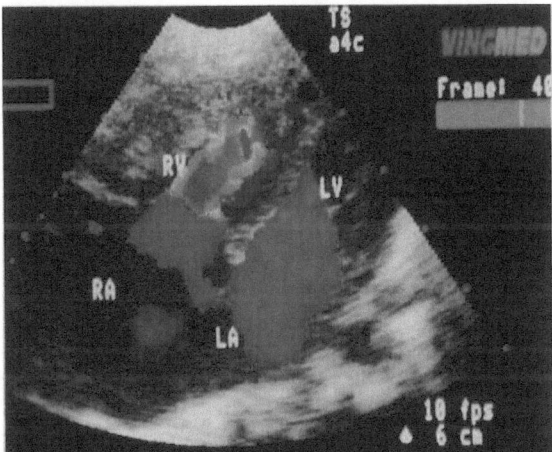

Fig. 6.81 Tricuspid stenosis in the apical four chamber view (RBG2). Narrowing of the tricuspid orifice at the upper left side of the mitral orifice shows aliasing as a sign of increased right ventricular inflow velocities at the valve level. See also the right-to-left shout on atrial level *(blue)*

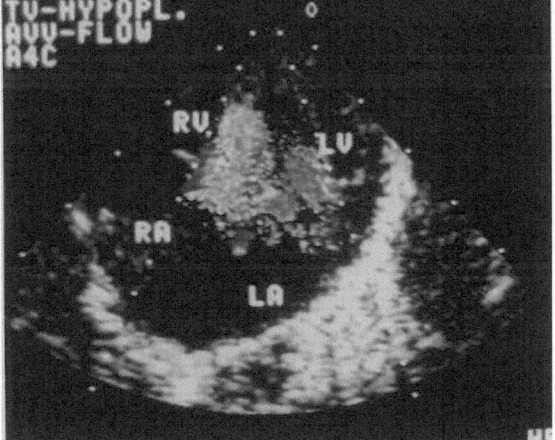

Fig. 6.82 Hypoplasia of the tricuspid orifice in univentricular heart in the apical four-chamber view, (RBG2). The inflow velocities across the tricuspid orifice are higher than through the mitral orifice, which is indicated by the brighter color on the *right side* of the heart

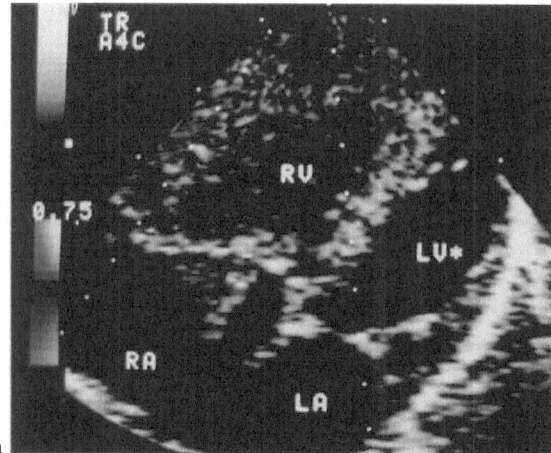

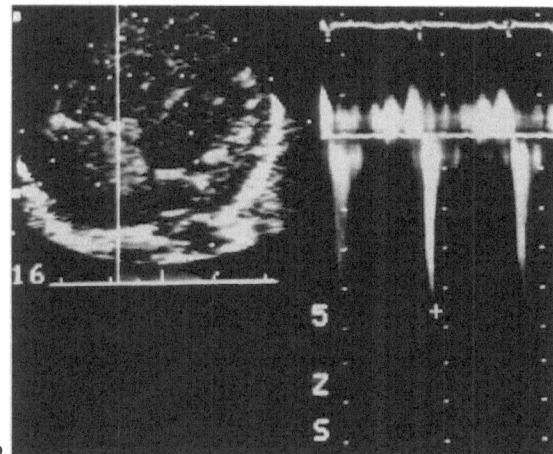

Fig. 6.83 a, b Very mild incompetence of an unaffected tricuspid valve (RBG2).
a Small regurgitant jet in right atrium *(RA)*, apical four-chamber view

b Continuous wave Doppler proves that tricuspid regurgitation is in this case indeed protosystolic and reaches various peak velocities

left side indicating increased flow velocities which are, however, below the level of aliasing (92 m/s in this case).

6.6.2 Tricuspid Regurgitation. Tricuspid regurgitation is a common finding in healthy individuals. Fig. 6.83 shows such an example: a narrow-based jet flows into the right atrium in early systole and extends posteriorly half way to the free wall. The M/Q-mode (see Fig. 5.14b, p. 37) suggests that the regurgitation is found only in early systole. This may, however, be a wrong impression because the jet may change its position as a result of the systolic motion of the heart and may, therefore, no longer be registered by the M/Q-line. That this assumption is not always true is indicated by the continuous wave Doppler trace in Fig. 6.83b. The beam diameter of the continuous wave Doppler is much larger than the M/Q-line and the fact that the regurgitation is observed only during early systole is considered to

Fig. 6.84a, b Severe tricuspid regurgitation in Ebstein's anomaly. **a** Apical four-chamber view (RBG2). Convective acceleration in the right ventricle in front of the tricuspid valve, regurgitant blood *(turquoise with yellow)* is filling nearly the entire length of the right atrium *(RA)*

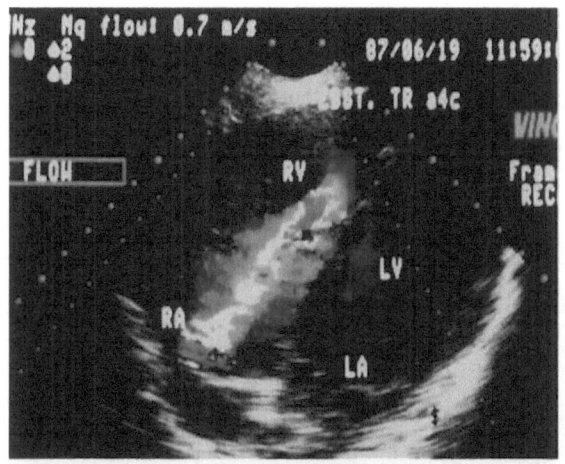

b M/Q-mode in the inferior cava (RB2). Holosystolic backflow *(red)* is caused by the severe regurgitation

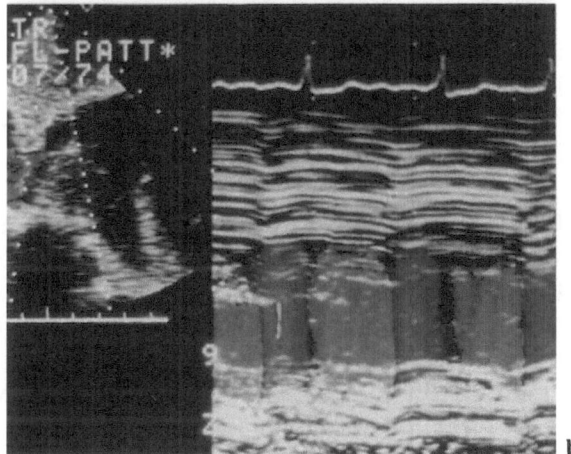

be the proof. *Innocent* tricuspid incompetence may also be holosystolic. Tricuspid regurgitation of *organic* origin is found, for instance, in Ebstein's anomaly, as shown in Fig. 6.84a. The regurgitant jet (cyan with yellow mosaic) can be seen to fill the complete length of the right atrium. In such severe tricuspid incompetence, systolic backflow into the inferior caval vein and the hepatic veins can be observed (Fig. 6.84b) and studies using contrast echocardiography have been reported earlier [34]. It has proved to be valuable in grading tricuspid regurgitation [41, p.57]. Measuring the maximal velocity of the regurgitant jet is a reliable method to determine right ventricular systolic pressure [40]. In some cases where the jet takes an atypical direction, CBFI has been proved to be helpful in aligning the continuous wave beam with the jet direction to obtain accurate results.

Diagnostic pitfalls may occur if the reflection of the inflowing systemic venous blood at the tricuspid valve in late systole is mistaken for tricuspid

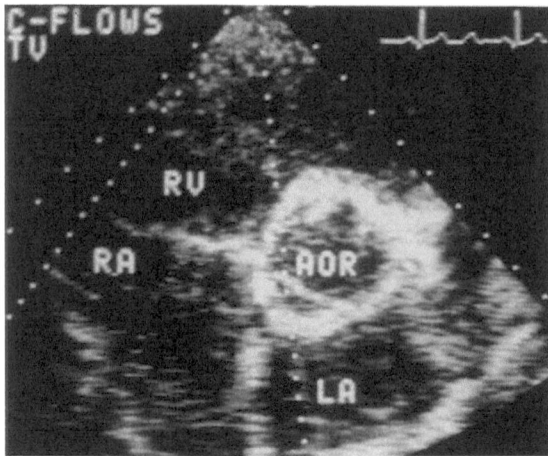

Fig. 6.85 Reflection *(blue)* of inflowing blood from the superior caval vein *(red)* at the closed tricuspid valve in late systole, parasternal short axis view. The aortic valves are still in an open position but outside the color sector. See text for more details

incompetence. This is shown in Fig. 6.85 where the venous inflow of the inferior caval vein in the right atrium can be seen in yellow-red. It is reflected from the septal leaflet of the tricuspid valve and appears in blue as it flows back into the right atrial cavity.

6.6.3 Tricuspid Valve Abnormalities in Complex Heart Disease. Tricuspid valve abnormalities in complex heart disease may consist of a *straddling* of the valve, as shown in Fig. 6.86. This figure shows in the apical four-chamber view that the tricuspid valve orifice is shifted to the left in relation to the upper rim of the ventricular septum. This causes the right atrium to empty partly into the left ventricle, the right ventricle is filled across the large VSD in a retrograde fashion (blue).

Atresia of the tricuspid valve is another abnormality which is always part of a complex cardiac malformation. In Fig. 6.87 it can be seen that the systemic venous blood bypasses the atretic tricuspid valve by an ASD which allows unimpeded right-to-left shunt (blue). Together with the pulmonary venous blood, it enters the ventricle across the mitral valve orifice thus causing relative mitral stenosis as indicated by the central aliasing. This figure shows two important pieces of information: first, the tricuspid valve is completely atretic and not just highly stenotic. Secondly, the ASD is large enough not to cause *any* obstruction to the shunt from right to left.

Tricuspid incompetence of organic origin is found, for example, in endocardial cushion defect and is shown in Fig. 6.88. Two regurgitant jets can be seen to originate at the closed tricuspid leaflets in systole and to extend into the right atrium (cyan with yellow mosaic), additionally there is right-to-left shunting across the primum atrial septal defect.

Fig. 6.86 Flow across a straddling tricuspid valve in the apical four-chamber view. RB2 mode has been selected for better discernibility of flow from cardiac structures. It is clearly shown that right atrial *(RA)* blood is entering the left ventricle *(LV)* because of the straddling of the tricuspid valve orifice above the ventricular inlet septum

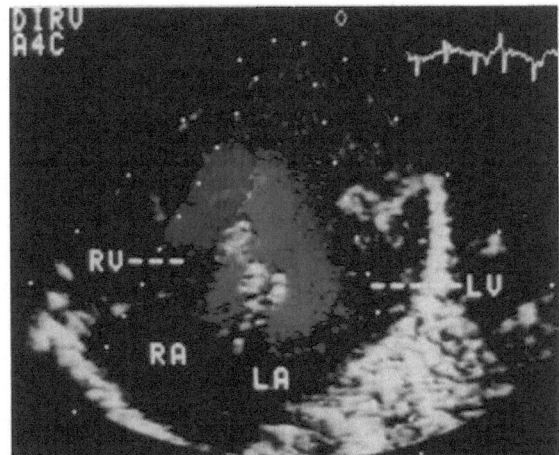

Fig. 6.87 Atresia of the tricuspid valve in the apical four-chamber view (RBG2). Systemic venous blood is flowing from the right atrium *(RA)* across an atrial septal defect into the left atrium *(LA)* and entering the ventricles across the mitral orifice together with the pulmonary venous blood, thereby causing high flow velocities in the mitral orifice, indicated by aliasing. See text for more information

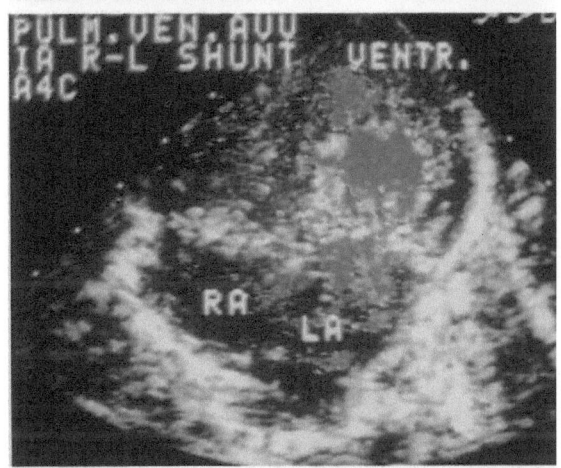

Fig. 6.88 Tricuspid incompetence in endocardial cushion defect across a cleft in the tricuspid valve, apical four-chamber view (RBG2). Two regurgitant jets *(cyan with yellow mosaic)* can be seen to originate at the tricuspid valve in systole *(1, 2)*, additionally there is right-to-left shunt across the primum atrial septal defect *(blue)* into the left atrium (LA)

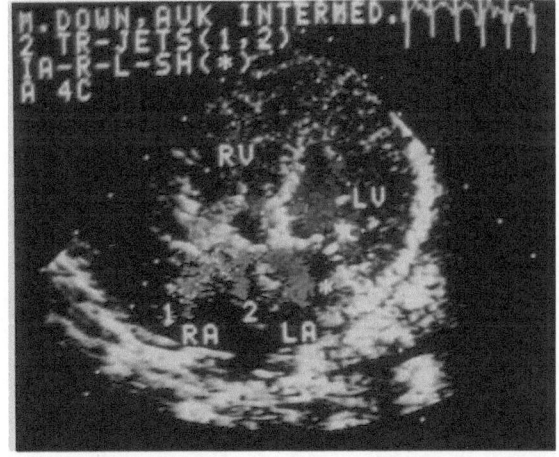

6.7 Abnormalities of the Right Ventricular Outflow

Obstruction of right ventricular outflow may occur at valvular level, it may be subvalvular or situated at the branching of the main pulmonary artery.

6.7.1 Pulmonic Valve Stenosis. Valvular pulmonic stenosis causes the blood to cross the narrowed pulmonary valve in a turbulent jet-like manner. In mild stenosis the jet is broad based and shows little aliasing (Fig. 6.89), in more severe obstruction of the pulmonic valve the jet diameter decreases and the amount of aliasing within the jet increases. In this condition the MPA exhibits considerable poststenotic dilatation which leads to streamline separation at the inferior wall [83] as indicated by the large yellow-red areas in Fig. 6.89. This phenomenon will be discussed in more detail in section 6.7.7. In severe pulmonic valve stenosis, dilatation

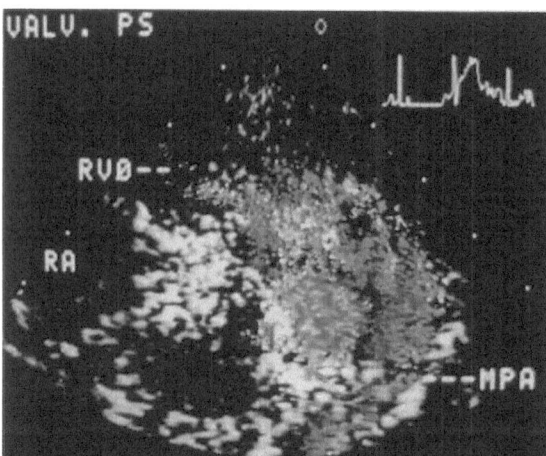

Fig. 6.89 Mild pulmonic valve stenosis, parasternal long axis view of the pulmonary artery in the sagittal plane (RBG2). A broad-based turbulent jet can be seen to originate at the pulmonic valve, the turbulence is indicated by the *cyan color speckled by yellow mosaic*. The *red-yellow area* at the lower border of the pulmonary artery is caused by backflowing blood induced by streamline separation (see section 6.7.7). At the bottom of the picture MPA can be seen to continue into the left branch

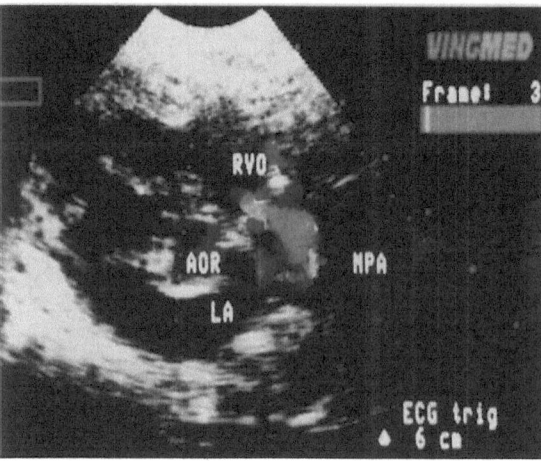

Fig. 6.90 High-degree pulmonary valve stenosis (RBG2). The jet has a very narrow base at the valve orifice and is imaged in a severe turbulent flow pattern. The poststenotic dilatation and the backflow area are less pronounced than in Fig. 89. This is a typical finding in severe pulmonic stenosis. The vibrations of the stenotic valve leaflets are displayed in red

Fig. 6.91 Right ventricular outflow *(RVO)* tract and proximal main pulmonary artery *(MPA)* in pulmonic stenosis, viewed from a low parasternal position in the sagittal long axis view (RBG2). Normal flow patterns in the right ventricular outflow can be seen to accelerate towards the narrowed pulmonary valve distal from which aliasing and turbulence are imaged as well as streamline separation *(red-yellow)*

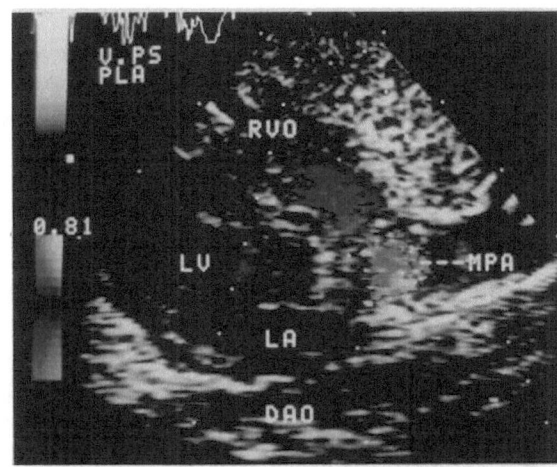

Fig. 6.92 High-volume flow in the pulmonary artery in a child with atrial and ventricular septal defects and complete atrioventricular block, parasternal long axis view in the sagittal plane (RBG2). *Mosaic flow pattern* is seen across the entire lumen of the pulmonary artery and is caused by the high-flow state (maximal displayable velocity: 92 m/s). There is, however, no jet formation and no backflow which helps to differentiate this flow condition from valvular pulmonic stenosis

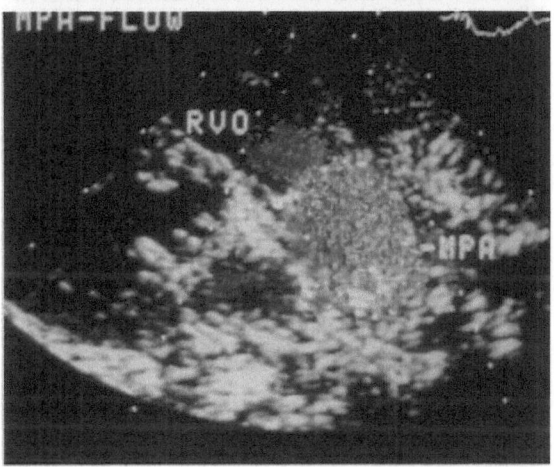

of the MPA is less pronounced (Fig. 6.90) leading to less marked streamline separation. The jet velocity is much higher, as indicated by multiple aliasing. Using a lower parasternal transducer position than that shown in Figs. 6.89 and 6.90, i. e., the fourth to fifth intercostal space in the parasternal position, allows a more detailed imaging of the subvalvular part of the right ventricular outflow tract, as shown in Fig. 6.91. Here turbulence, aliasing, and streamline separation can be seen to occur in the MPA in pulmonic valvular stenosis. Blood flow in the right ventricular outflow tract is, however, completely undisturbed, indicating that the stenosis is entirely valvular. Fig. 6.89 also demonstrates that flow disturbances induced by pulmonic stenosis extend mainly into the left branch.

Diagnostic pitfalls may be caused in high-flow states in the pulmonary artery. Fig. 6.92 shows such an example in which left-to-right shunt across an ASD and a VSD together with complete atrioventricular block lead to a very high stroke volume of the right ventricle with subsequent relative pulmonary stenosis. From the flow image, however, it is evident that flow disturbances take place over the entire diameter of the pulmonary artery in the same fashion, and that no jet formation or streamline separation appear (in contrast to Figs. 6.89 and 6.90).

6.7.2 Subpulmonic Stenosis. Subpulmonic stenosis often accompanies valvular pulmonic stenosis in its isolated form or is combined with other cardiac malformations. Fig. 6.93 shows an example of pulmonary stenosis with subvalvular obstruction in the subcostal long axis view of the right ventricular outflow. Flow abnormalities are indicated by aliasing and appear proximal to the pulmonic valve in the distal outflow tract extending across the valve into the MPA. In a case of hypoplastic infundibulum Fig. 6.94 demonstrates a case of subpulmonic obstruction in *tetralogy of*

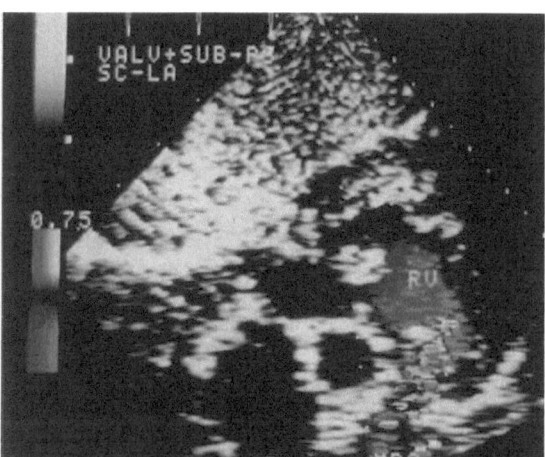

Fig. 6.93 Localized subpulmonary stenosis secondary to valvular pulmonic stenosis, subcostal long axis view of the right ventricular outflow tract *(RVO)* (RBG2). Morphological systolic narrowing of the right ventricular outflow can be found to cause flow disturbances proximal to the pulmonic valve (see Fig. 6.91 for comparison)

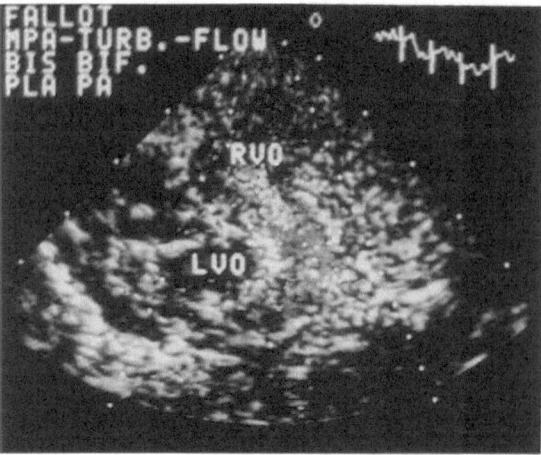

Fig. 6.94 Hypoplastic infundibulum in tetralogy of Fallot, parasternal long axis view in the sagittal plane (RBG2). Turbulent flow can be seen to extend all along the narrowed right ventricular outflow tract *(RVO)* and is more pronounced here than in the pulmonary artery pointing out that the main obstruction to pulmonary blood flow is due to infundibular hypoplasia

Fig. 6.95 Pulmonary artery banding in an infant with multiple ventricular septal defects, parasternal long axis view. CBFI demonstrates acceleration towards the banding site with aliasing proximal to artificial stenosis. The distal part of the pulmonary artery *(PA)* exhibits only a little coloration which points towards an effective result of the banding

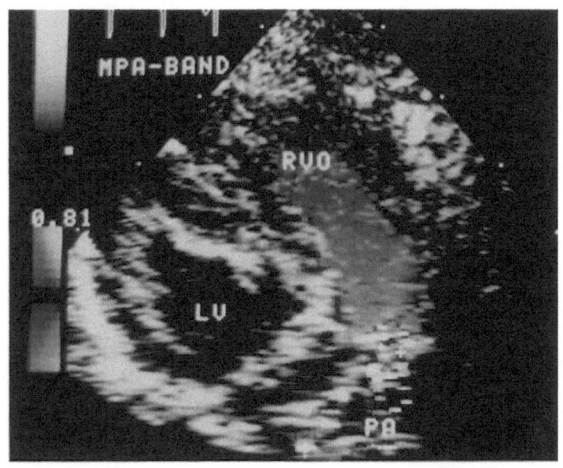

Fallot in which flow disturbances can be seen all along the narrow right ventricular outflow tract.

6.7.3 Banding of Pulmonary Artery. Banding of the pulmonary artery is still an important surgical method for the effective treatment of infants in congestive heart failure because of multiple VSDs or complex shunt lesions [70]. In Fig. 6.95 systolic flow in the pulmonary artery can be seen to accelerate towards the banding and to pass across it in a highly turbulent manner. There is much less coloration in the pulmonary artery distal to the banding, which indicates, in our experience, an effective narrowing by the band.

6.7.4 Pulmonary Valve Atresia. In pulmonary valve atresia the anterograde blood flow from the right ventricle into the pulmonary artery is completely absent. The perfusion of the pulmonary arterial system is therefore dependent on the patency of the ductus arteriosus and/or the existence of bronchial collateral vessels. In Fig. 6.96 an example of pulmonary atresia with intact ventricular septum is shown in a neonate. This systolic frame demonstrates normal systolic outflow into the aortic root in contrast to which the pulmonary artery (to the right of the blue left ventricular outflow) does not show any signs of blood flow. The ductus arteriosus seems to be very narrow or even closed. There is considerable tricuspid regurgitation (cyan-yellow mosaic in the right atrium) which represents the only way in which blood can leave the right ventricle in systole.

6.7.5 Branching Stenosis of the Pulmonary Artery. Branching stenoses of the pulmonary artery can be considered to be normal in the first weeks of life (see p. 40). After the age of 3 months they represent pathological find-

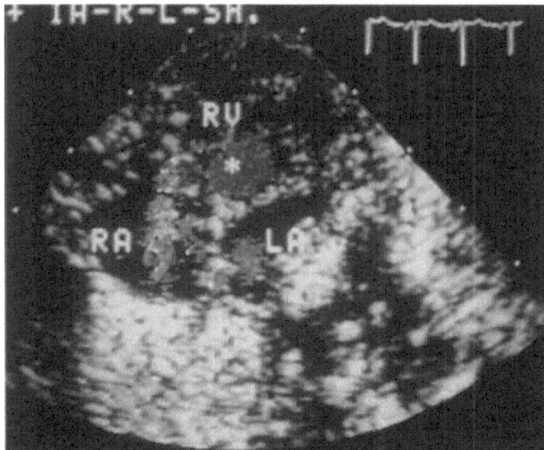

Fig. 6.96 Pulmonic valve atresia with intact ventricular septum, parasternal short axis view (RBG2). Normal outflow of the left ventricle is shown by *blue coloration* of left ventricular outflow tract (asterisk), no signs of significant blood flow in the pulmonary artery (at *the right side* of left ventricular outflow) are detectable, nor does the right ventricle *(RV)* show any significant coloration towards the outflow. Instead, tricuspid regurgitation *(cyan with yellow mosaic)* is the only systolic outflow from the right ventricular cavity

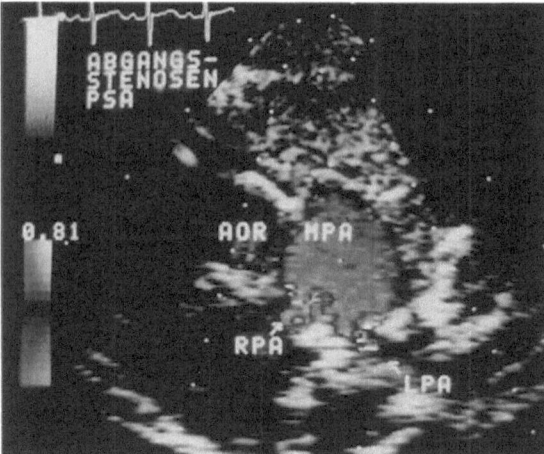

Fig. 6.97 Bilateral branching stenoses of pulmonary artery, viewed in the parasternal short axis view of the base, in a child with Alagille syndrome (RBG2). Convective acceleration towards the narrowed branches can be seen to occur at both sides of the bifurcation (indicated by *aliasing* and *mosaic pattern*)

ings, as shown in Fig. 6.97 in a child of 1⅓ years of age with an Alagille syndrome and bilateral stenoses. A unilateral stenosis on the right side with a pressure drop of about 20 mmHg as determined by continuous wave Doppler is shown in Fig. 6.98. In branching stenoses the combination of CBFI and continuous wave Doppler is especially valuable because the investigations beam can be aimed directly at the area of turbulence.

6.7.6 Pulmonary Valve Incompetence. Pulmonary regurgitation is frequently found in normal individuals [19, p. 111]. In slight degrees the regurgitation can be seen only proximal to the pulmonary valve in the right ventricular outflow tract (Figs. 6.99 a, 6.100 b) and appears holodiastolic in most cases (Fig. 6.99 b). Sometimes two jets can be imaged (Fig. 6.100 b).

In more severe forms of pulmonic valve incompetence the regurgitant flow velocities already have considerable values in the MPA, which is

Fig. 6.98 Unilateral branching stenosis of the right side, same view as Fig. 6.97 (RBG2 with determination of systolic gradient by continuous wave Doppler). CBFI allows the precise alignment of the continuous wave beam *(dotted line)* with the stenosis imaged by CBFI. The maximal systolic gradient is 20 mmHg

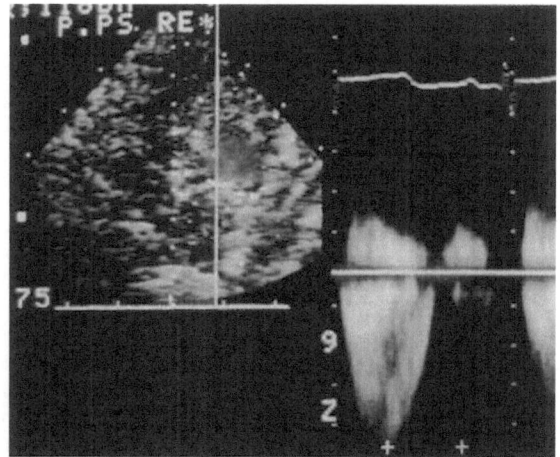

Fig. 6.99 a, b Slight degree of pulmonic regurgitation with normal pulmonary artery pressure (RBG2).
a A small *yellow jet* in the right ventricle *(RV)* extending from the pulmonic valve indicates slight incompetence

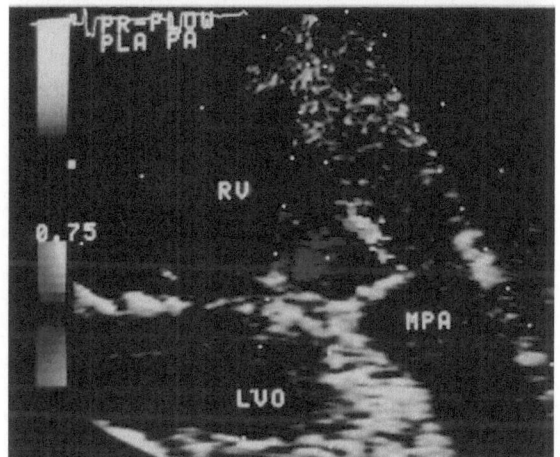

b M/Q-mode displays holodiastolic timing of incompetence *(red-yellow),* normal systolic outflow is displayed in *blue*

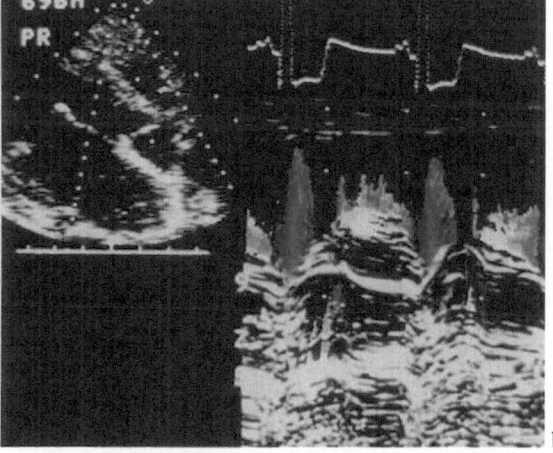

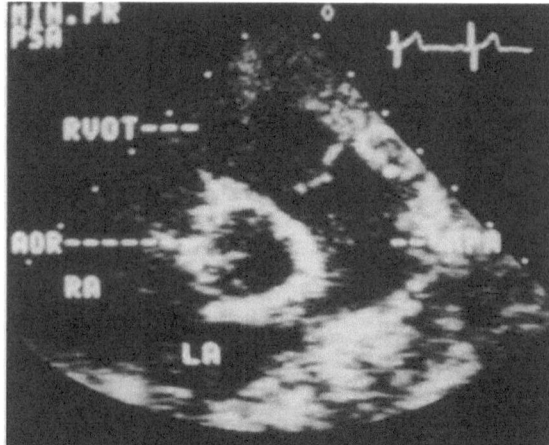

Fig. 6.100a, b Moderate pulmonic regurgitation viewed in the parasternal short axis plane.
a The 2D echocardiograph shows a diastolic gap between the free edges of the posterior and one of the anterior valve leaflets

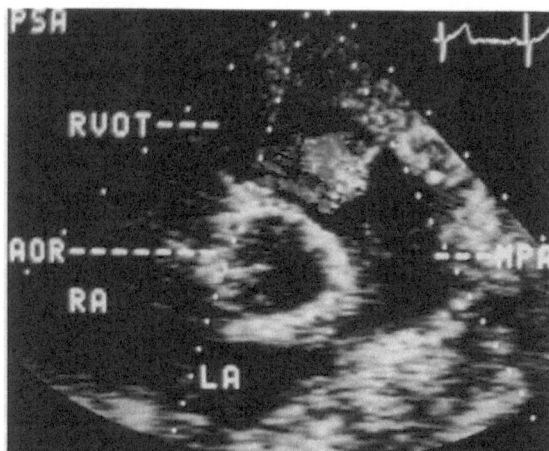

b Superposition of CBFI reveals moderate incompetence of the pulmonary valve, in addition to the expected jet a second one is imaged which seems to originate outside the 2D plane

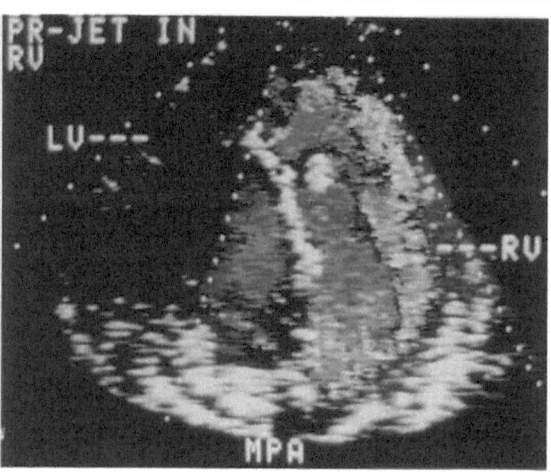

Fig. 6.101 Severe pulmonary regurgitation in congenital aplasia of the pulmonic valve, subcostal long axis view of the right ventricular outflow (RBG2). The regurgitant jet extends down into the right ventricle *(RV)* below the anterior papillary muscle, causing forward-flow towards the valve. Additionally, diastolic turbulence can be seen to occur in the main pulmonary artery *(MPA)*

shown in Fig. 101. It is our experience that this always indicates some pathological condition (i.e., pulmonary hypertension or organic pulmonary valve disease). A method for grading pulmonary regurgitation with the use of CBFI has been proposed [29] and consists of determination of the pulmonary regurgitation index area by planimetry and standardization by body surface area.

In normal diastolic pressure conditions in the pulmonary artery, the diastolic backflow does not show any aliasing (Figs. 6.99, 6.100b). In pulmonary hypertension, however, regurgitant velocities exceed the Nyquist limit which causes aliasing or even diastolic turbulence (Fig. 6.101) to appear.

6.7.7 Systolic Flow Reversal. Systolic reversal of flow direction in the pulmonary artery was described by our group as a sign of pulmonary hypertension in 1980 using single-gate pulsed Doppler [54]. It consists of a backflow towards the right ventricular outflow tract localized distal to the posterior pulmonic valve (Fig. 6.102) and it has subsequently been proved to be valuable for the detection and evaluation of pulmonary hypertension [51, 52]. This flow phenomenon of systolic flow reversal can be described more accurately using CBFI [82] and seems to be responsible for the mesosystolic notching of the pulmonary valve [80, 83, 84]. Early in systole, outflow into the MPA exhibits normal flow distribution across the entire area of the vessel, as is shown in Fig. 5.20b (p. 40). A little later, however, a considerable part of the pulmonary artery at the inferior wall is occupied by blood flowing towards the transducer (Fig. 6.102, 2D insert). At the supe-

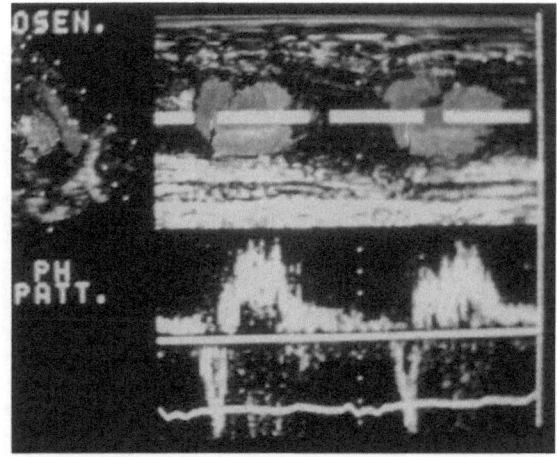

Fig. 6.102 Systolic flow reversal displayed in all modes of pulsed Doppler display (RBG2). CBFI *(upper left)* in a child with pulmonic vein stenoses is frozen in late systole and shows a considerable area of backflow towards the posterior pulmonary valve leaflet. The M/Q-line runs through this backflow area *(dotted line),* the sample volume of the single gate Doppler is positioned on this line distal to the posterior leaflet *(I).* The M/Q-mode *(upper right)* demonstrates short anterograde *(blue)* and considerable retrograde *(red-orange)* flow time which lasts into early diastole. The single gate Doppler trace presents the same information at one point in the conventional manner of display

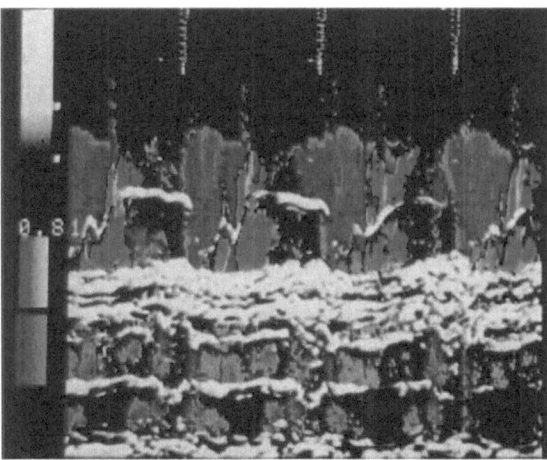

Fig. 6.103 M/Q-mode recorded distal to the posterior pulmonary leaflet in a patient with idiopathic ectasia of the pulmonary artery (RBG1). The motion of the posterior leaflet is displayed in *white on black* and the flow vectors are displayed in the usual coloration. From this trace (especially the second systole) it is evident that systolic notching and flow reversal are occurring at the same time

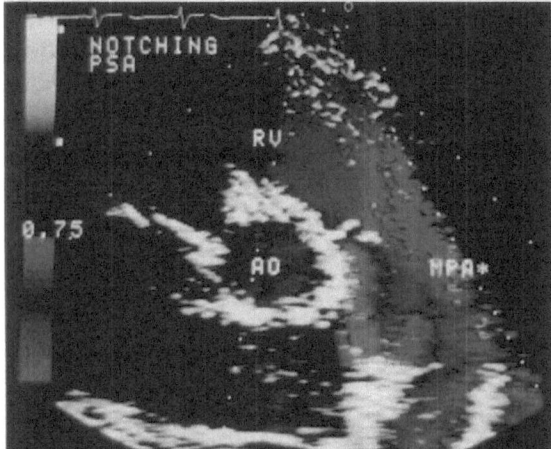

Fig. 6.104 a, b Subsequent frames of pulmonary valve motion and flow conditions in an ectatic pulmonary artery (RB2).
a A small part of the posterior leaflet near the wall has been moved into a closed position by systolic backflow occupying a small area of pulmonary artery in the second third of systole. The residual part of the leaflet is still held in an open position by the orthograde blood flow. The red area at the *upper (right)* margin is caused by aliasing

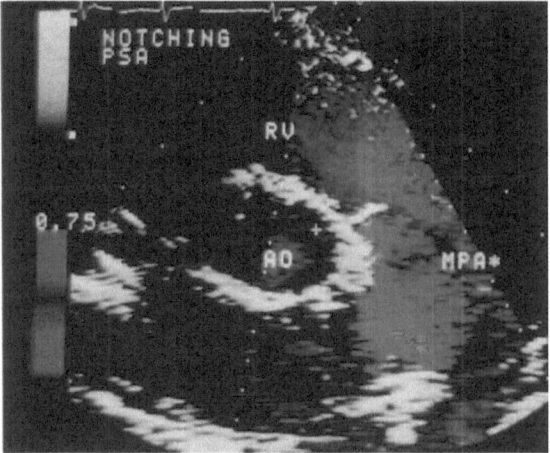

b The whole posterior leaflet has been moved into the closed position by the increasing amount of backflowing blood in the last third of systole. See text for more details

rior wall blood is still flowing from the right ventricle into the pulmonary artery exhibiting even higher velocities than before, as indicated by central aliasing. In Fig. 6.103 the M/Q-mode was recorded near the inferior wall of the pulmonary artery, from this it is evident that the systolic notching of the pulmonic valve occurs at the same time as the backflow towards the valve and is therefore the cause of the former as the valve moves only passively with the blood stream. Fig. 6.104 shows that the systolic closing motion of the pulmonic valve is an event which is not carried out by the whole valve at once, as in the case of physiological end-systolic closure. Rather, the posterior leaflet moves gradually into the mid-systolic closing position, starting at the anulus and being pushed more and more into the orifice as the backflowing volume increases.

Like the notching phenomenon, systolic flow reversal is not specific for pulmonary hypertension [2] but may be found in a variety of conditions [84]. The common denominator to all these conditions is a considerable dilatation of the MPA [84] which causes streamline separation (see p. 23).

6.7.8 Pulmonary Valve Abnormalities in Complex Heart Disease. Pulmonary valve disease in complex heart disease is relatively common and consists in most cases of pulmonic valve stenosis or atresia. One of the morphological signs of *transposition of the great arteries* is the parallel course of the great arteries at their origin from the ventricles. If there is additional pulmonic stenosis, the posterior vessel shows systolic turbulence, as can be seen from Fig. 6.105. Fig. 6.106a shows a comparatively small vessel below and in front of the much larger descending aorta with a systolic immobile valve in a neonate with *tricuspid atresia*. Fig. 6.106b demonstrates that systolic outflow (blue) does not continue into this vessel which is therefore obviously the pulmonic artery with an atretic valve.

Sometimes high-degree *pulmonic stenosis* in indistinguishable from *pulmonic valve atresia* with conventional echocardiographic means. In such cases CBFI may help to clarify the situation by displaying the flow pattern in the MPA, as demonstrated in Fig. 6.107. It shows the time distribution of flow in the aortic root and the hypoplastic MPA which is continuously perfused by the PDA. Additionally, flow disturbances appear in systole (blue mottling) which are obviously caused by anterograde flow across the stenotic valve.

Aplasia of the pulmonic valve is caused by the congenital absence of the pulmonary valve. Instead, an irregular slight rim of primitive connective tissue is present at the expected area of the valve [11]. The pulmonic valve itself is hypoplastic. The hemodynamic consequences of this malformation is a stenotic and, at the same time, a severely incompetent pulmonic valve. In most cases, a combination with a VSD is found. In our experience, CBFI is very useful in describing the pathological flow situation found in

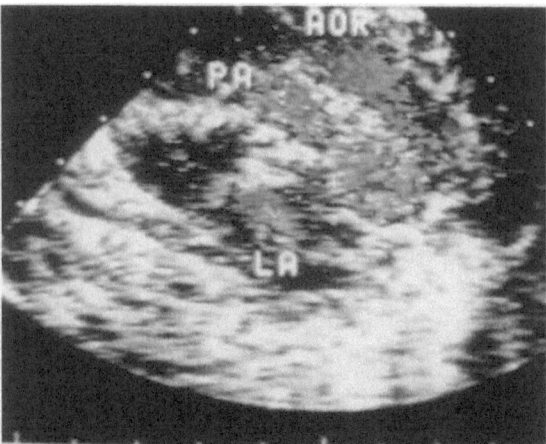

Fig. 6.105 Parallel course of the great arteries in congenitally corrected transposition of the great arteries (L-TGA), parasternal long axis view of the arteries (RBG2). Turbulent flow *(mosaic pattern)* in the posterior vessel helps to identify this as pulmonary artery (with valvular stenosis)

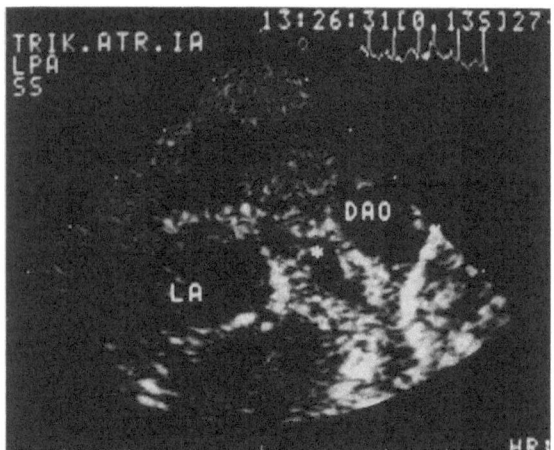

Fig. 6.106a, b Pulmonary valve atresia in tricuspid atresia with normal origin of the great arteries, suprasternal view.
a A hypoplastic artery is shown *below* and *in front of* the descending aorta *(DAO)* with an immobile valve *(asterisk)*

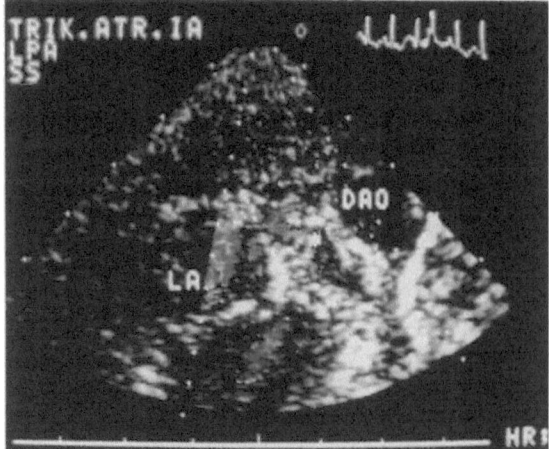

b Superpositioning of CBFI reveals atresia of the valve, as indicated by the fact that flow *(blue)* in the hypoplastic right ventricular infundibulum does not continue across the atretic valve into the pulmonary artery (RBG2)

Fig. 6.107 M/Q-mode of pulmonary artery flow in a neonate with high-degree pulmonic stenosis and tricuspid atresia (RB2) reveals systolic turbulence *(blue)* intermingling with the continuous systolic-diastolic blood flow into the pulmonary artery across the patent ductus *(red)*

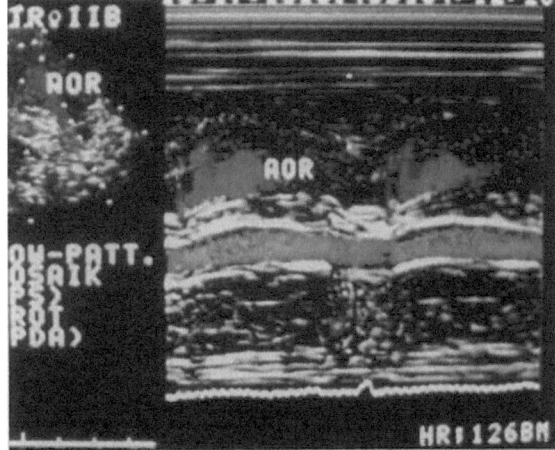

Fig. 6.108a, b Right pulmonary artery near the bifurcation in aplasia of the pulmonary valve, suprasternal view.
a Severe dilatation is visible in the 2D echocardiogram

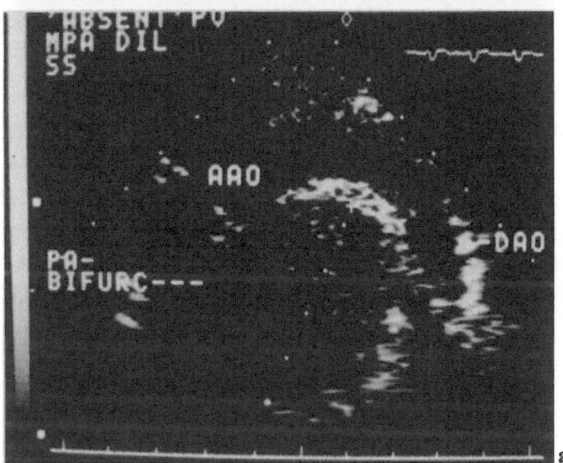

b Adding CBFI identifies flow disturbances across the entire lumen of the right pulmonary artery

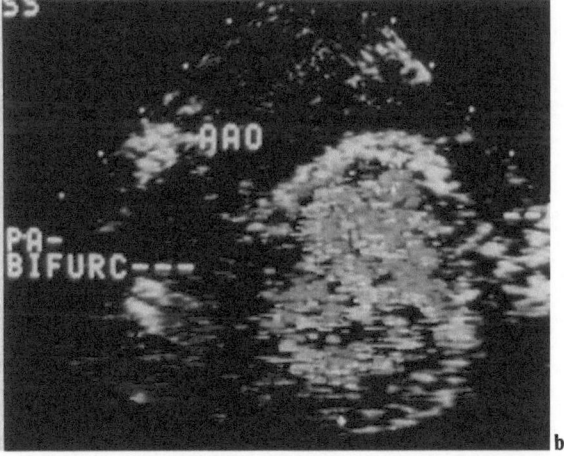

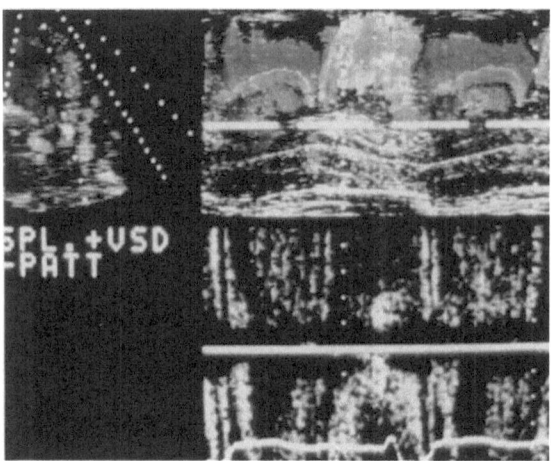

Fig. 6.109 Severe flow disturbances in the right ventricular outflow tract in aplasia of the pulmonic valve (RBG2). CBFI *(upper left)* shows severe diastolic regurgitation *(red-orange)*. The M/Q-line *(dotted)* runs along the outflow tract into the pulmonary artery. M/Q-mode displays systolic *(arc-like aliasing)* and diastolic flow disturbances at the valve orifice, single gate Doppler trace shows the conventional display which is much more difficult to understand than the M/Q-mode in this case

the MPA in this situation. Fig. 6.108a shows an unusually large right pulmonary artery near the bifurcation, viewed from the suprasternal position, which exhibits severe systolic flow disturbances filling the whole lumen (Fig. 108b). Fig. 6.109 demonstrates the severely disturbed systolic flow and pulmonic regurgitation at the valvular level. In systole there is threefold aliasing at the maximally displayable velocity of 69 cm/s, which means a peak velocity of more than 180 cm/s. Additionally, severe pulmonic regurgitation is demonstrated in the M/Q-mode, Doppler trace, and 2D flow image.

References

1. Abbasi AS, Allen MW, De Cristofero D, Ungar I (1980) Detection and estimation of the degree of mitral regurgitation by range-gated pulsed Doppler echocardiography. Circulation 61: 143
2. Baumann W, Wann LS, Childress R, Weyman AE, Feigenbaum H, Dillon JC (1979) Midsystolic notching of the pulmonary valve in the absence of pulmonary hypertension. Am J Cardiol 43: 1049
3. Baylen BG, Meyer RA, Kaplan S (1975) Echocardiographic assessment of severity of patent ductus arteriosus with pulmonary disease. J. Pediatr 86: 423
4. Bierman FZ, Williams RG (1979) Subxyphoid two-dimensional imaging of the interatrial septum in infants and neonates with congenital heart disease. Circulation 60: 80
5. Bommer WJ, Miller L (1982) Real-time two-dimensional color-flow Doppler: enhanced Doppler flow imaging in the diagnosis of cardiovascular disease. Am J Cardiol 49: 944
6. Bouchard A, Yock PG, Schiller NB, Newlands JS, Massi BM, Botvinick EH, Greenberg B, Cheitlin MD (1985) Quantitation of chronic aortic insufficiency using color Doppler flow mapping. Circulation 72 [Suppl III]: 100
7. Brandestini M (1978) Topoflow – a digital full range Doppler velocity meter. IEEE Trans Son and Ultrason SU-25: 287
8. Byard EC, Perry GJ, Roitman DI, Nanda NC (1985) Quantitative assessment of aortic regurgitation by color Doppler. Circulation 72 [Suppl III]: 146
9. Davis RA, Feigenbaum H, Chang S, Konecke CC, Dillon JC (1974) Echocardiographic manifestations of discrete subaortic stenosis. Am J Cardiol 33: 277
10. Edwards JE, Burchell HB (1958) Pathologic anatomy of mitral insufficiency. Proc Mayo Clin 33: 497
11. Emmanouilides GC, Baylen BG (1983) Congenital absence of the pulmonary valve. In: Adams FH, Emmanouilides GC (eds) Heart disease in infants, children and adolescents, 3rd ed. Williams and Wilkins, Baltimore, p 228
12. Estevez CN, Dillon JC, Walker PD, Feigenbaum H, Chang S (1976) Echocardiographic manifestations of aortic cusp rupture in a case of myxomatous degeneration of the aortic valve. Chest 69: 544
13. Feigenbaum H (1970) Echocardiography. 2nd ed. Lea and Febiger, Philadelphia, p 174
14. Feigenbaum H (1986) Echocardiography. 4th ed. Lea and Febiger, Philadelphia
15. Forfar JC, Godman MJ (1985) Functional and anatomical correlates in atrial septal defect. Br Heart J 54: 193
16. Fujioka T, Ueda K, Ohkawa S, Kamata C, Kitano K, Ito J, Takahashi R, Shinagawa T, Matsushita S, Sugiura M, Murakami M, Hada Y (1978) A clinicopathological study of aortic regurgitation with septal fluttering on echocardiogram. J Cardiogr 8: 697
17. Gittenberger-De Groot AC (1977) Peristent ductus arteriosus: most probably a primary congenital malformation. Br Heart J 39: 610
18. Graham TP, Bender HW, Spach MS (1983) Ventricular septal defect. In: Adams FH, Emmanouilides GC (eds) Heart disease in children, infants and adolescents. Williams and Wilkins, Baltimore, p 134
19. Hatle L, Angelsen B (1985) Doppler ultrasound in cardiology, 2nd ed. Lea and Febiger, Philadelphia, p 111

20. Henry WL, de Maria A, Gramiak R, King DL, Kisslo JA, Popp RL, Sahn DJ, Schiller NB, Tajik A, Teichholz LE, Weyman AE (1980) Report of the American Society of Echocardiography Committee on nomenclature and standards in twodimensional echocardiography. Circulation 62: 212

21. Henzi M, Burckhardt D, Raeder EA, Follath F (1976) Echocardiography as a method for the determination of the severity of aortic insufficiency. Schweiz Med Wochenschr 106: 1557

22. Heymann AM (1983) Patent ductus arteriosus. In: Adams FH, Emmanouilides GC (eds) Heart disease in infants, children and adolescents. Williams and Wilkins, Baltimore, p 158

23. Holen J, Simonsen S (1979) Determination of pressure gradient in mitral stenosis with Doppler echocardiography. Br Heart J 41: 529

24. Hsiung MC, Zachariah ZP, Nanda NC, Roitman DI (1985) Color Doppler assessment of mitral regurgitation induced by supine exercise in ischemic heart disease. Circulation 72 [Suppl III]: 58

25. Jenni R, Vieli A, Ruffmann K, Krayenbühl HP, Anliker M (1984) A comparison between single gate and multigate ultrasonic Doppler measurements for the assessment of the velocity pattern in the human ascending aorta. Eur Heart J 5: 948

26. Kalmanson D, Veyrat C, Derai C, Savier CH, Berkmann M, Chiche P (1972) Non-invasive technique for diagnosing atrial septal defect and assessing shunt volume using directional Doppler ultrasound. Correlations with phasic flow velocity ₋atterns of the shunt. Br Heart J 34 (10): 981

27. Kirklin JW, Barat-Boyes BG (1986) Cardiac surgery. Wiley, New York, p 720

28. Kitabatake A, Ito H, Tanouchi J, Ishihara K, Fuji K, Joshida Y, Nakatani S, Kamada T (1985) A new approach to quantitate aortic regurgitation by real time two-dimensional Doppler echocardiography. Circulation 72 [Suppl III]: 306

29. Kobayashi J, Hirose H, Nakano S, Matsuda H, Kishimoto H, Kato H, Arisawa J, Kawashima Y (1986) Quantitative evaluation of pulmonary regurgitation after correction of tetralogy of Fallot by two-dimensional (real time color) pulsed Doppler echocardiography. In: Doyle EF, Engle MA, Geosouy WM, Rashkind WJ, Talner NS (eds) Pediatric cardiology. Springer, Berlin Heidelberg New York Tokyo, p 129

30. Kyo S, Omoto R, Takamoto S, Yokote Y (1984) Noninvasive analysis of bi-directional multiphasic intracardiac shunts by real-time-two-dimensional Doppler echocardiography. Circulation 70 [Suppl II]: 365

31. Kyo S, Omoto R, Takamoto S, Takanawa E (1984) Clinical significance of color flow mapping real-time two-dimensional Doppler echocardiography (2-D Doppler) in congenital heart disease. Circulation 70 [Suppl II]: 37

32. Lê TP, Redel DA (1985) Bestimmung des Links-Rechts Shunts bei Vorhofseptumdefekt vom Ostium secundum Typ mittels Farb-Doppler-Echokardiographie. Z Kardiol 74 [Suppl 5]: 78

33. Lê TP, Redel DA, Wippermann CF (1986) Erkennung von Ductusshunts und Abschätzung des Links-Rechts Shunts bei PDA mittels Farb-Doppler-Echokardiographie. Z Kardiol 75 [Suppl I]: 78

34. Lieppe W, Behar VS, Scallion R, Kisslo JA (1978) Detection of tricuspid regurgitation with two-dimensional echocardiography and peripheral vein injection. Circulation 57: 128

35. Machii K, Hirai H, Nishizawa S, Matsuzaki H, Suzuki M, Yamaguchi T, Kuvako K (1987) Detection of slow flow and disturbed flow patterns with power-mode and dispersion-mode 2D-color flow mapping. J Cardiovasc Ultrason, 4: 6

36. Marino P, Zanolla L, Perini GP, Salazzari GC, Conti F, Poppi A (1981) Critical assessment of two-dimensional echocardiographic estimation of the mitral valve area on rheumatic mitral valve disease - calcific deposits in the valve as a major determinant of the accuracy of the method. Eur Heart J 2: 197

37. Martin RP, Rakowski H, Kleiman JH, Beaver W, London E, Popp RL (1979) Reliability and reproducibility of two-dimensional echocardiographic measurement of the stenotic mitral valve orifice area. Am J Cardiol 43: 560

38. Namekawa K, Kasai C (1984) Principle and equipment. In: Omoto R (ed) Color atlas of real-time two-dimensional Doppler echocardiography. Shindau-To-Chiryo, Tokyo, p 5

39. Namekawa K, Kasai C, Tsukamoto M, Koyano A (1982) Imaging of blood flow using autocorrelation. Ultrasound Med Biol 8: 138

40. Nishimura RA, Tagik A (1986) Measurement of intracardiac pressures - state of the art. Herz 11: 283

41. Omoto R (1984) Acquired valvular disease. In: Omoto R (ed) Color Atlas of Real-time two-dimensional Doppler echocardiography. Shindau-to-Chiryo, Tokyo
42. Omoto R, Yokote Y, Takamoto S, Kyo S, Ueda K, Asano H, Namekawa K, Kasai C, Kondo J, Koyano A (1984) The development of real-time two-dimensional Doppler echocardiography and its clinical significance in acquired valvular disease. With specific reference to the evaluation of valvular regurgitation. Jpn Heart J 25: 325
43. Otsuji Y, Tei C, Kisanuki A, Arikawa K, Kawazoe Y, Kagoshima K, Tanaka H (1985) Assessment of the change of mitral regurgitant volume flow by colour Doppler echocardiography. Circulation 72 [Suppl III]: 306
44. Perloff JK (1970) The clinical recognition of congenital heart disease. Saunders, Philadelphia, p 333
45. Prandtl L, Oswatitsch K, Wieghardt K (1984) Führer durch die Strömungslehre, 8th edn. Vieweg, Braunschweig
46. Pyerik RE, Wappel MA (1983) Mitral valve dysfunction in the Marfan syndrome. Am J Med 74: 797
47. Quinones MA, Young JB, Waggoner AD, Ribeiro LGT, Miller RR (1980) Assessment of pulsed Doppler echocardiography in detection and quantification of aortic and mitral regurgitation. Br Heart J 44: 612
48. Rashkind WJ, Miller WW (1966) Creation of an atrial septal defect without thoracotomy: a palliative approach to complete transposition of the great arteries. J Am Med Assoc 196: 991
49. Redel DA (1982) How to investigate aorta and pulmonary artery in congenital heart disease. In: Peronneau P, Baker DW, Diebold B (eds) Cardiovascular applications of Doppler echocardiography. Inserm 111: 541
50. Redel DA (1985) Angeborene Herzfehler im Kindesalter. Befunde der zweidimensionalen und Doppler-Echokardiographie. In: Grube E (ed) Zweidimensionale Echokardiographie. Thieme, Stuttgart, p 290
51. Redel DA (1985) Hohlvenen, rechter Vorhof, rechter Ventrikel und Arteria pulmonalis. In: Grube E (ed) Zweidimensionale Echokardiographie. Thieme, Stuttgart, p 96
52. Redel DA, Fehske W (1984) Diagnosis and follow-up of congenital heart disease in children with the use of twodimensional Doppler echocardiography. Ultrasound Med Biol 10: 249
53. Redel DA, Jünck H (1985) Description of blood flow velocity profiles inside the human main pulmonary artery with the use of color Doppler echocardiography. J Cardiovasc Ultrason IV: 4
54. Redel DA, Viëtor S (1980) Pulsed Doppler echocardiography – a non-invasive technique for assessment of pulmonary hypertension in children. World Congr Ped Cardiol, London, 1980
55. Reid GE, Cortes LE, Claus RH, Reppert EH (1970) The surgical repair of duplication of the mitral orifice. Am Thorac Surg 9: 81
56. Reuben SR, Swadling JP, de Lee G (1970) Velocity profiles in the main pulmonary artery of dogs and man, measured with a thin-film resistance anemometer Circulation Res 27: 995
57. Riemenschneider TA (1983) Left ventricular-right atrial communication. In: Adams FH, Emmanoulides GC (eds) Heart disease in infants, children and adolescents, 3rd edn. Williams and Wilkins, Baltimore, p 154
58. Robertson WS, Stewart J, Armstrong WF, Dillon JC, Feigenbaum H (1984) Reverse doming of the anterior mitral leaflet with severe aortic regurgitation. J Am Coll Cardiol 3: 431
59. Rudolph A (1974) Congenital diseases of the heart. Year Book Medical Publishers, Chicago, p 37
60. Sahn DJ, Allen H (1979) Real-time cross-sectional echocardiographic imaging and measurement of the patent ductus arteriosus in infants and children. Circulation 58: 343
61. Satomi G, Takao A, Momma K, Mori K, Audo M, Tonyama K, Konishi T, Tomimatsu H, Nakazawa M, Nakamura K (1986) Detection of the drainage in anomalous pulmonary venous connection by two-dimensional Doppler color flow-mapping echocardiography. Heart Vessels 2: 41
62. Satomi G, Nakazawa M, Takao A, Mori K, Tonyama K, Konishi T, Tomimatsu H. Nakamura K (1986) Blood flow pattern of the interatrial communication in patients with complete transposition of the great arteries: a pulsed Doppler echocardiographic study. Circulation 73: 95
63. Sellers RD, Levy MJ, Amplatz K, Sillehei CW (1964) Left retrograde cineangiocardiography in acquired cardiac disease: technique, indication and interpretation in 700 cases. Am J Cardiol 14: 437

64. Shapiro JN, Martin RP, Fowles RE, Popp RL (1979) Single and twodimensional echocardiographic features of the interatrial septum in normal subjects and patients with an atrial septal defect. Am J Cardiol 43: 816
65. Shinebourne EA, Anderson RH (1980) Current paediatric cardiology. Oxford University Press, Oxford, p 21
66. Silverman NK, Levin AB, Heyman MA, Rudolph A (1974) Echocardiographic assessment of ductus arteriosus shunt in premature infants. Circulation 50: 821
67. Skjaerpe T, Hatle L (1981) Diagnosis and assessment of tricuspid regurgitation with Doppler ultrasound. In: Rijsterborgh H (ed) Echocardiology. Nijhoff, The Hague, p 299
68. Smallhorn JF, Huhta JC, Adams PA, Anderson RH, Wilkinson JL, MacCartney FJ (1983) Cross-sectional echocardiographic assessment of coarctation in the sick neonate and infant. Br Heart J 50: 349
69. Spirito R, Baron BJ (1984) Pattern of systolic anterior motion of the mitral valve in hypertrophic cardiomyopathy: assessment of two-dimensional echocardiography. Am J Cardiol 54: 1039
70. Stark J (1983) Pulmonary artery banding. In: Stark J, de Leval M (eds) Surgery for congenital heart defects. Grune and Stratton, London, p 187
71. Takamoto S (1984) Pitfalls in reading: artifact signals. In: Omoto R (ed) Color atlas of realtime two-dimensional Doppler echocardiography. Shindau-To-Chiryo, Tokyo, p 29
72. Toguchi M, Ichimiya S, Yokoi K, Hibi N, Kambe T (1981) Clinical investigation of aortic insufficiency by means of pulsed Doppler echocardiography. Jpn Heart J 22: 537
73. Van Praagh R, McNamara JJ (1968) Anatomic types of ventricular septal defect with aortic insufficiency: diagnostic and surgical considerations. Am Heart J 75: 604
74. Varghese PJ, Izukawa T, Celermajer J, Simon A, Rowe RD (1969) Aneurysm of the membraneous ventricular septum. A method of spontaneous closure of small ventricular septal defect. Am J Cardiol 24: 531
75. Veyrat C, Cholot N, Abithol G, Kalmanson D (1980) Non-invasive diagnosis and assessment of aortic valve disease and evaluation of aortic prosthesis function using echo pulsed Doppler velocimetry. Br Heart J 43: 393
76. Veyrat C, Lessana A, Abitbol G, Ameur A, Benaim R, Kalmanson D (1983) New indexes for assessing aortic regurgitation with two-dimensional Doppler echocardiographic measurement of the regurgitant aortic valvular area. Circulation 68: 998
77. Ward JM, Baker DW, Rubenstein SA, Johnson SL (1977) Detection of aortic insufficiency by pulsed Doppler echocardiography. J Clin Ultrasound 5: 5
78. Weyman AE (1982) Cross-sectional echocardiography. Lea and Febiger, Philadelphia, p 212
79. Weyman AE, Caldwell RL, Hurwitz RA, Girod DA, Dillon JC, Feigenbaum H, Green D (1978) Cross-sectional echocardiographic detection of aortic obstruction. 2. Coarctation of the aorta. Circulation 57: 498
80. Weyman AE, Dillon JC, Feigenbaum H, Chang S (1974) Echocardiographic patterns of pulmonary valve motion with pulmonary hypertension. Circulation 50: 905
81. Wharton MJ, Nesmith JW, Shaw MC, Kisslo J (1985) Normal Doppler color flow map patterns of the left ventricular outflow tract imitating aortic insufficiency. Circulation 72 [Suppl III]: 100
82. Wippermann CF, Redel DA (1985) Description of main pulmonary artery flow reversal in pulmonary hypertension with color Doppler echocardiography. J Cardiovasc. Ultrasound 4: 26
83. Wippermann CF, Redel DA (1986) The mechanism of the mesosystolic "notching" of the pulmonic valve revealed by Doppler-flow-imaging. Circulation 74 [Suppl II]: 132
84. Wippermann CF, Redel DA (1987) Die Dilatation der Arteria pulmonalis mit konsekutiver Strömungsablösung als Erklärung der mesosystolischen Schließbewegung der Pulmonalklappe. Herz Kreisl 19: 91
85. Wippermann CF, Redel DA, Bremer D (1987) Noninvasive estimation of the right ventricular pressure in patients with VSD by color-Doppler directed continuous wave Doppler and the blood pressure. Eur J Pediatr 146: 100
86. Wranne B, Ask P, Loyd D (1986) Quantification of heart valve regurgitation by jet intrusion. In: Cardiac Doppler, vol II. Spencer MP (ed) Nijhoff, Dordrecht, p 133
87. Yoshida J, Funabashi T, Nakaya S, Maeda T, Taniguchi N (1980) Subxiphoid cross sectional echocardiographic imaging of the "goose neck" deformity in endocardial cushion defect. Circulation 62: 1319

Subject Index

Numbers in bold type indicate pages upon which the subject is treated extensively